THE BEER DIET

How to Drink Beer and NOT Gain Weight

GARY GREENBERG

The Beer Diet
How to Drink Beer and Not Gain Weight

For information, contact the author at:
SuperWriterInc@gmail.com

Published by Cosmic Café Press • Boca Raton, Florida

ISBN: 978-0-578-71295-6

Cover illustration and design:
Jason Robinson / robinzson@aol.com

Back cover photo: Tom DiPace

The book is designed to provide helpful information on the subjects of beer and health. It is not meant to be used, nor should it be used, to diagnose or treat any medical condition. For diagnosis or treatment of any medical condition, consult a healthcare provider. The publisher and author bear no responsibility for any specific health or allergy needs for anyone reading or following the suggestions in this book. The physicians and other people mentioned in this book have not endorsed any of the information or recommendations offered. Any references are provided for informational purposes only and do not constitute endorsement of any products, websites or other sources.

For Nora and Glen, who on many occasions saved my life by fetching me a beer

&

For all of the rugby players and beer-lovers in the world

Author's Note

This book is not intended to promote, encourage or condone alcohol abuse. The scientific evidence is clear that drinking too much of any alcoholic beverage, including beer, is bad for health and longevity. However, the reality is that a shitload of people overindulge, and we know from Nancy Reagan's 1980s-era anti-drug campaign, telling them to "just say no" doesn't work. I sincerely hope that illuminating the dangers of alcohol in these pages will make at least some drinkers think twice about their consumption of it. But if people are going to drink a lot of beer, they can compensate to some degree by otherwise taking good care of their bodies. I offer suggestions on how to do that and potentially lessen beer's impact on their weight and general health. These ideas come from my own personal experience as well as research I have done over the years as natural health journalist. *The Beer Diet* has not been evaluated by medical professionals, including the ones quoted in the following pages. So take it for what it's worth to you.

Table of Contents

Preface
The Original Beer Diet

I first heard about a beer diet from my brother Rick. He was a coxswain on the Dartmouth College rowing team back in the early 1970s. The coxswain is the little guy who sits in the stern of the shell. His main tasks are to pace the oarsmen by pounding out a rowing beat with a block of wood against the side of the shell while also steering the craft, and then getting thrown into the water when they win. Like horse-racing jockeys, it's important for coxswains to be as close to the 110-pound minimum weight as possible, because the less weight the oarsmen have to propel through the water, the faster the shell will go.

Rick was actually the second-team coxswain. The first-teamer was John Eaton, the wiry grandson of a noted industrialist. Eaton had a big personality and the devil-may-care attitude towards life you often find in kids from wealthy families. Some of his exploits at Dartmouth border on legendary, and there are many stories about him I'm sure he'd rather not see in print, including one that involved a flooded gas station bathroom and toilet seat souvenir.

But Eaton always seemed very proud of his beer diet. Despite his naturally lean physique, he still had to drop weight to get close to the 110-pound mark. He accomplished this by consuming nothing but beer from Thursday mornings until after the Saturday afternoon races. That not only reduced his calorie intake but reversed it, as previously consumed solid foodstuffs found their way out of his body and, best case scenario, into a nearby commode. The liquid sustenance also acted as a diuretic, ridding his body of whatever excess fluids that were left through his bladder and colon.

After two-plus days on his beer diet, Eaton invariably lost the requisite weight. More remarkably, he still managed to steer the shell straight, a feat he attributed to his Irish heritage.

Although Eaton's beer diet helped catapult him to the national team, I wouldn't recommend it to anyone (with the possible exception of Irish coxswains). However, I must point out that beer is a fairly healthy concoction. It's common knowledge that in medieval times, people, even kids, drank beer instead of water because it was less likely to be contaminated by bacteria, parasites, raw sewage and other nasty stuff.

Well, maybe not.

Like a lot of common knowledge, that little tidbit of popular history is not entirely true. There were plenty of clean water sources in the Middle Ages, and the people of that era were also enlightened enough to boil drinking water if necessary.

Still, beer was viewed as a more nutritious alternative to water, and farmers and other workers imbibed in the calorie-laden drink to slake their thirst and provide a boost of energy during sun-up-to-sun-down jobs. Beer also supplies several essential nutrients. And, believe it or not, scientific studies suggest that moderate consumption of beer can help reduce the risk of cancer, heart disease, diabetes, kidney and gall stones, high blood pressure, osteoporosis, cataracts, dementia and various infections, as well as tight-ass dancing.

Despite its numerous health benefits, man cannot live on beer alone. Even John Eaton knew this, as he spent at least four days a week sustaining his bodily functions with sustenance in addition to beer. And what you eat when you're not drinking beer (or along with it), has a lot to do about how well you can maintain a reasonable weight and still enjoy tipping back a few pints.

So *The Beer Diet* is actually a game plan for how beer-lovers can achieve this goal, even in a world with an ever-increasing selection of high-calorie, high-carb craft beers. Imagine downing twenty or so beers a week and still fitting into pants with a thirty-two-inch waist. I've been doing it for years and am happy to share my secrets with you.

After all, who wants to drink alone?

Everything in moderation, including moderation.

--Oscar Wilde, Irish writer and namesake of a mild ale from Mighty Oaks brewery in Essex, England

Chapter 1
The Beer Diet

The first time my lips tasted beer was in June of 1968 on the East Bank of the Chesapeake Bay in Maryland. My family had a thirty-six-foot Pacemaker cabin-cruiser on the Sassafras River, and we used to tie up with a half-dozen or so other boats to hang out in a cove by Knight Island, which is actually a peninsula. I was almost fifteen and wearing a plaster cast from hip to toes as my broken femur continued to mend from a February car accident. So while my brothers and friends were out waterskiing, I was stuck with the adults as they enjoyed some end-of-day cocktails on Dolly and Nat Neuman's houseboat.

I sequestered myself on the stern of our boat, looking out towards Chesapeake Bay. A narrow, padded bench stretched from rail to rail and was the most comfortable spot for me as I could rest my casted right leg on it and lean back on a pile of cushions.

I heard Dolly Neuman shout, "Don't worry, I'll get it," and watched her amble across the sterns of the three boats between hers and ours with a kind of tipsy feline grace.

She saw me and announced: "Ran out of scotch. Need another bottle."

When she got to our boat, I expected her to head straight for the nook where my parents kept the booze. But instead, she came my way.

"How ya doin'?" she asked.

I smiled flatly. "OK, I guess." She could tell I was a little deflated, so she plopped down on the other end of the bench and started chatting away.

Dolly was my mom's best friend and very glamorous looking, with coifed hair and long fake eyelashes that she wore even on the boat. Bathing suits were pretty conservative back then, but they were better than clothes as far as a pubescent boy was concerned, and Dolly was well put together for a mom. She was also a little looped. I don't remember most of what we talked about, but I do remember imagining that she was Mrs. Robinson from *The Graduate,* and I was the graduate.

As Dolly yakked away about various things, I focused on her dancer's legs and cleavage. She was nice and funny and a straight-shooter, saying things most adults wouldn't say to a kid.

"So I told Flo and Sam, 'If you want to have sex on the boat, you should at least close the front hatch,'" she said with a laugh.

Dolly squinted in a funny way when she laughed. We used to say she looked like a Chinaman, though you can't really say that anymore. Maybe Asian. In any case, I'd imitate her, which made her laugh harder and squint even more, at which point I'd squint more, and so on through a couple of rounds.

After a few minutes of banter, she said, "Well, they're gonna be wondering if I fell overboard or something. I better head on back to my boat."

I nodded and thanked her for taking time away from the cocktail party to talk to me.

"Hey," she said as she stood up. "You want a beer?"

I shrugged. "I dunno. Maybe." Dolly winked one of her heavily-lashed eyes, then grabbed a handle of Dewar's White Label and teetered off. Everybody cheered when she arrived with the scotch. In a minute or two, she came back with a bottle of Miller High Life.

"Here," she said, handing it to me. "It's the champagne of bottled beer," she added with another squinty-eyed laugh. "Don't tell your mother I gave it to you."

With that, she traversed the little flotilla back to her houseboat, *Happy Talk*. When she got there, I heard her say something, and a round of laughter erupted. Adults definitely had more fun when they were drinking.

It was getting close to sunset. The river was smooth as glass, the best time to waterski. I sighed and took a sip. The beer was kind of warm and absolutely the worst thing I'd ever tasted. I tried another sip, then leaned over the transom and poured the rest into the river, apologizing to the fish.

That Was Then, This Is Now

I still have no taste for Miller High Life, but I never forgot Dolly's compassion in taking time from a rousing good cocktail party to keep a temporarily crippled young teen company, fuel his sexual fantasies and give him his first beer.

There have been many since then. As a longtime rugby player, drinking a lot of beer kind of goes with the territory. You need a bit of anesthetizing after playing a high-impact game without pads. Beer didn't seem to affect my weight much when I was young, but when I hit my mid-forties I started putting on a pound or two a year. A decade later, I'd gained nearly twenty pounds and could no longer fit into my size 32 rugby shorts. Compounding the problem, I got swept up in the craft beer craze. I even started brewing my own and now drink near a case a week of the potent, high-calorie stuff. Yet here I am in my mid-sixties, still playing rugby and once again a trim size 32.

This book explains how I did it, and continue to do it. Since you are not me, doing exactly what I have done may or may not work as well for you. But, hopefully, you will at least be inspired to do something. Because if you don't and get too fat, it is likely to trigger a cascade of health issues that will eventually have your doctor telling you to cut down or even eliminate your beer consumption. And nobody wants that. Use the tips and insights I've gleaned from years of being a beer-loving natural health writer to develop your own plan, so you, like me, can continue to enjoy drinking plenty of your favorite beverage without gaining weight.

A Beer Renaissance

For those of you who may have skipped the Preface of this book, let me reiterate that The Beer Diet™ (not really) is not a matter of drinking beer and consuming nothing else, though the concept is intriguing. On a beer-only diet, you would lack a certain amount of vital nutrients to maintain peak health, despite the fact that beer does contain vitamins, minerals and antioxidants, not to mention a fair measure of carbohydrates, which you don't really need but are hard to avoid. Beer also contains alcohol, which is basically a poison, but fun. It's the alcohol in beer that gives you that warm, fuzzy feeling that all is right in the world when it is really quite screwed up. A little alcohol is actually good for you, but a lot will hurt you a lot. The debate, as always, is how much is a little, and how much is a lot? The American Medical Association's guidelines say two drinks a day for men and one for women is okay. I doubt that's really okay with most women, who in the Age of #MeToo no doubt want an equal opportunity to get warm and fuzzy feelings. Although it may be a party killer, the AMA warns that exceeding those guidelines raises risk of all kinds of maladies, ranging from heart disease to cancer to diabetes to dementia, not to mention car wrecks, firearm accidents and White supremacy movements.

Sadly, the destructive nature of the demon alcohol is what most limits us when indulging in this wonderful delicacy, which many of my personal friends (primarily rugby players) would drink most of the time, if they don't already. But as I polish off a bottle of Dogfish Head 90 Minute Imperial IPA, 9 percent alcohol by volume (ABV), I decide that it is way too early in the book to bum everyone out. So we'll pick up this discussion later on.

In any case, why should the beer mug be viewed as half-empty? Beer is an incredible beverage. Born before wine, whiskey and bread, it has outlasted every major civilization on Earth since before there even were major civilizations on Earth. And in this day and age (Tuesday, Post-Millennium) we are blessed to be in the midst of a Beer Renaissance. With breweries of all sizes popping up everywhere from Ashville to Zionsville, the art of brewing the foamy delight continues to reach new heights, and varieties, like Funky Buddha's Maple Bacon Coffee Porter.

While some imbibers are purists in preferring beer made with only malt, hops, yeast and water, others enjoy the exploding trend of culinary-influenced ales, which include relatively exotic ingredients, such as those in Funky Buddha's much admired specialty ale, presumably made with maple syrup and coffee (they are very secretive about the actual ingredients but admit they use smoked malt and spices to get the bacon flavor). A former homebrewer named Ryan Sentz came up with that recipe when the Funky Buddha was just a storefront hookah lounge in a strip mall in sleepy Boca Raton, Florida. The Maple Bacon Coffee Porter, so-called "Roadside Diner Breakfast in a Glass," gained global cult status, enabling Sentz to open up a warehouse-sized brewery and tap room in the Oakland Park section of Fort Lauderdale. It's still there, and so is Sentz on occasion, even though he and his brother KC sold out to beverage giant Constellation Brands, Inc., for an "undisclosed figure" that was reputed to be well north of $100 million.

I met Ryan Sentz once and still have his business card. Along with beer and hookah tobacco, the Funky Buddha Lounge in Boca Raton sold homebrew supplies and, as a homebrewer myself, I needed some specialty grains and yeast for an upcoming batch. I will discuss the agonies and ecstasies of homebrewing in a later chapter. Suffice to say for now that it is a fun and rewarding pastime, so long as your beer bottles don't explode. It can be so much fun that my wife Nora and I came up with the brilliant idea of planning beer-brewing parties. We figured them to be something like Tupperware parties but with the focus shifting from plastic storage containers to what is not-even-arguably Planet Earth's best beverage ever.

So anyway, when I met Ryan Sentz in the Funky Buddha homebrew section, he mentioned that he was opening up a bigger brewery in Fort Lauderdale. I told him about Tupperware-style homebrewing parties. He at least pretended to be interested. The key, I explained, would be to work out a deal with a guy like him to get a piece of the action from anyone I enticed into homebrewing and sent to him for supplies (basically a non-virtual associate's program). He continued to humor me by giving me his card and saying, "Let me know how it goes."

Of course, it didn't go anywhere because, like most people, my wife and I are better at coming up with brilliant ideas than actually executing them.

A Very Brief History Of Beer

Before I got distracted by Funky Buddha's Maple Bacon Coffee Porter, I was waxing poetic about mankind's timeless devotion to beer. You have to wonder how someone came up with the idea in the first place. No one really knows when beer was first created, although one school of Biblical brew scholars insists that after making the heavens and earth and all living things in six days, God kicked back with a flagon of ale on the seventh.

It's likely that humans discovered beer around the same time we began cultivating crops, including barley, in the Fertile Crescent some 12,000 years ago. Historians figure that the Neolithic farmers must have left harvested grain out in the rain, and it was eventually fermented by wild yeast. Just like today, back then there must have been one joker nutty enough to do something really stupid for a laugh, like drinking tainted barley rainwater. It probably tasted pretty nasty, but no doubt the buzz from the alcohol was worth it, especially in an era when there wasn't really much else to do for entertainment.

There is evidence that the Sumerians were brewing beer 6,000 years ago, as a tablet (clay, not iPad) depicts a crowd using reed straws to drink beer from a communal bowl, which was kind of like a primitive keg party. By 1800 B.C., the Sumerians worshipped a Goddess of Brewing named Ninkasi, and an ode to her (also written on a clay tablet) includes the oldest beer recipe ever found:

Ninkasi, you are the one who soaks the malt in a jar…You are the one who spreads the cooked mash on large reed mats…You are the one who holds with both hands the great sweet wort you place appropriately in a large collector vat...When you pour out the filtered beer of the collector vat, it is like the onrush of Tigris and Euphrates.

Nearly 4,000 years later, Fritz Maytag, founder of Anchor Brewing in San Francisco, actually made a "Ninkasi Beer" based on that recipe. Lacking bittering hops, it reportedly tasted more like hard apple cider than beer and had an ABV of 3.5 percent, which is roughly equivalent to Old Milwaukee Light.

But all of that, except for Maytag and Old Milwaukee Light, is ancient history and thus has nothing to do with how a 21st century rugby player and other beer-lovers can imbibe in their favorite beverage without piling on the pounds. So without further ado, we will begin to address that issue in the next chapter.

Chapter 2
The Beer Belly Myth

It's common knowledge that people who drink a lot of beer get a beer belly. It's a bulbous midriff protuberance, which seems to affect men more than women and, ironically, can make them look somewhat pregnant. Anybody with eyes and an aging friend or relative or co-worker who likes to drink a lot of beer is probably familiar with this phenomenon. It's plain as day, except to some nitpicking scientists who actually measure - rather than eyeball - such things. They insist that beer is not the primary reason people get beer bellies. While this is hard to believe, it is good news for us.

To really understand why beer itself doesn't cause beer bellies, you have to understand exactly what beer is. In another writer's hands, this could be really boring, like a passage from my SAT reading comprehension test back in high school. It was a very dense four- or five-paragraph treatise on brewing beer, with no mention of things like Maple Bacon Coffee Porter or rugby players standing on their heads to chug beers, an impressive, if senseless, display of athletic prowess.

Back in high school, I wasn't really interested in beer. I was more interested in girls, like the two Nancys who sat on either side of me in math class. I let them cheat off of me during tests, hoping that one or both would show some romantic interest in me. They didn't, but at least they were nice to me (especially right before tests), which wasn't normally the case with the kind of girls I would have liked to date. You see, before I started drinking beer, I was a runty little guy who was often picked on and never got the girl. After starting to drink beer, I filled out a bit, put my bully-tempered toughness to good use by taking up the sport of rugby, and got some choice girls to take an interest in me despite the fact that I was still somewhat of a runt.

Coincidence? I think not.

What Beer Is

Getting back to business, here's what beer is: water, malted grain (traditionally barley), hops and yeast. Of course, renegades like Ryan Sentz add various other foodstuffs to their brews, but that overcomplicates the issue. And in Germany, where beer is called *bier* and has been made since at least the Weihenstephan Abbey was licensed to produce the stuff in 1040, there is a beer purity law (Reinheitsgebot) forbidding anything that contains ingredients other than water, barley, hops and yeast to be labeled as "bier." For simplicity's sake, we will focus on these basic ingredients and how they may, or may not, promote the phenomenon known as a beer (or bier) belly.

Water: While man needs water to live, he can't live on it alone. That's because water is the original zero-calorie drink, and you need calories to fuel your body. If you drink too much water, your belly may swell, but your body will quickly absorb what it needs and eliminate the excess. The really good news for us is: Beer is close to 95 percent water. So, in a way, almost all of the beer we drink has no calories. We really only need to worry about the other 5 percent, at least as far as promoting both subcutaneous and visceral fat in and about the abdomen, aka, a beer belly.

Of course, we do need to consider the water itself. While it may have no fat-spawning calories, your typical tap water often has toxins like chlorine, fluoride, lead, mercury and even arsenic, not to mention a variety of pharmaceutical drugs that have been carelessly discarded and worked their way back into the drinking water supply. Government regulators consistently insist there are only "harmless" traces of these substances, but you've got to wonder how much they add up over the course of decades when you consider we probably consume more water, in one form or another, than anything else on Earth.

You may think that a substance like chlorine is harmless because it is put into swimming pools to protect your health. And while it may keep you from getting things like an ear infection or brain-eating amoeba, it is a poison. Chlorine kills any and all microorganisms. In gaseous form, it's been used by despots like Saddam and Assad to annihilate great swaths of their own people. So immerse your body in it if you must (although the skin may seem waterproof to you, it is really more like a sponge), but I definitely wouldn't advise drinking it.

Fluoride is another one. Most people think putting fluoride into our drinking water was a good idea because it helps to prevent cavities. Others aren't so sure. While I don't believe, like some, that the fluoridation of our water was a communist plot (it started well before Putin's reign), I do believe the undisputed fact that fluoride is a neurotoxin, meaning it kills brain cells. And we really want to maintain as many brain cells as possible because they come in handy to remember things, like beer recipes. Fluoride is also an endocrine disruptor, meaning it wreaks havoc on hormones, particularly those of the thyroid and pineal glands. Since the thyroid gland's hormones regulate metabolism, screwing them up can result in weight gain, among other things, and possibly contribute to a beer belly. As a writer, I personally have never liked fluoride because for decades before spell-check was developed, I always spelled it "flouride."

Tap water may also contain lead, mercury, cadmium, arsenic, pharmaceutical drugs, PCBs, DDT, HCB and even MtBE… (I'd explain what all of these things are but promised I wouldn't bore you like the reading comprehension section of the SATs). It's all nasty stuff and you want to reduce your exposure as much as possible.

Fortunately, modern-day brewers typically purify the local water and then add minerals and other compounds back in to optimize the chemistry for whatever type of beer they are making. So the quality of the water is typically not relevant when choosing a fine ale to quaff (as opposed to things like taste, ABV and price). Besides that, you can't really control it, and this book only focuses on stuff you can control. In this case, you can control the rest of the water you consume. So go get yourself a reverse-osmosis filter for your drinking water at home. That way, most of what ends up inside of you will be free of contaminants. This type of strategy will be a recurring theme in this book: The smarter you are about your choices – some as easy as getting a reverse-osmosis water filter -- the more you can indulge in your favorite beverage.

To sum up: Water is a vitally important ingredient of beer, but not so much when it comes to beer bellies.

Malt: Of the four primary ingredients in beer, malt is the only one that has a direct impact on weight gain and the main reason that beer is sometimes called "liquid bread." It is relatively high in carbohydrates, which are sugars along with starches that mostly turn into sugars during the digestive process. We could talk about complex carbs and simple carbs but it doesn't really matter at this point.

For me, just hearing the word "malt" conjures up thoughts of those rich, delicious, waistline-be-damned malted milkshakes I used to get at my friendly neighborhood drugstore soda fountain in the days when drugstores actually had soda fountains. Like beer malt, the malt in those milkshakes was mostly made from barley (with a little wheat flour and evaporated milk thrown in). Malt for beer is created by soaking barley (or other grains) for a few days until it begins to germinate, then raising the heat to stop the germination process and dry out the grain. This process turns most of the starch in it into fermentable sugars with the help of an enzyme called diastase. But I can see that just mention of the word "enzyme" has your eyelids starting to droop, so I will dispense with any more chemistry.

The basic point is that malting produces sugar, and as we all know, sugar has a lot of calories. The blend of sugars in malted barley is mostly maltose with some glucose, sucrose and a dash of fructose thrown in. It is lower on the glycemic index (a scale of how fast sugars hit your bloodstream, and the lower the better) than commonly used white sugar and the ubiquitous high fructose corn syrup, but still has about 85 calories per ounce of weight. That's notable because, other than water, malt is the main ingredient in beer. To put it into perspective, in a typical five-gallon batch of homebrew, I add nine pounds of molasses-like liquid malt extract, compared to a few ounces of hop pellets and just grams of yeast powder.

The amount of sugars in barley malt become somewhat of a moot point when you consider that the fermentation process turns more than 90 percent of those sugars into alcohol. Obviously, the more fermentable sugars the malt contains, the more alcohol will ultimately be produced. And since it's still too early to talk much about alcohol without depressing everyone, we can turn to some of the many good things in malt.

Barley, in itself, is quite healthy. Some even call it a superfood, due to a type of dietary fiber that experts say can reduce risk of obesity, diabetes and heart disease, according to an article in the *Daily Mail*, a British tabloid that rarely gets everything right. No matter. Most if not all of that fiber gets lost as the grain is smashed, mashed and fermented. Still, what remains is rich in B vitamins, which are important in metabolizing the sugar, fat and protein you ingest, turning it into energy so it doesn't end up around your waist. It contains a sprinkling of amino acids that you need to make proteins, the so-called "building blocks of life." Malted barley has some antioxidants, which neutralize inflammation-inducing oxidative stress on a cellular level. It also has minerals such as potassium, phosphorus, calcium and magnesium, and it's one of the few dietary sources of silicon, which is necessary for bone health and may help protect against osteoporosis. Besides all of these wonderful things, it can make us happy. The compound hordenine found in malted barley activates the feel-good dopamine D2 receptor in the brain, according to scientists at Friedrich-Alexander-Universität Erlangen-Nürnberg in Germany, who are likely to be more reliable than *Daily Mail* "experts."

To sum up: Malts used for brewing have some carbs that ultimately could contribute to a beer belly, but also minerals, vitamins and other compounds that your body needs.

Hops: Hops are the yin to malt's yang. The bitter buds are used to balance the sweetness of the malt, and are most prominent today in "hop-forward" beers like India pale ales (IPAs). Hops were discovered by the Roman philosopher and naturalist Pliny the Elder, who died during the eruption of Mount Vesuvius in 79 A.D. and is perhaps best remembered by the modern beer community for having Russian River brewery's legendary Pliny the Elder Imperial IPA named after him. Even though beer was around in Pliny's day, it was typically bittered not by the newly discovered hops by rather by wild rosemary, heather, sweet gale, bog myrtle and other herbs, flowers and spices collectively called gruit. Then, in the 12th century, a Benedictine abbess named Hildegard of Bingen noted in her scientific treatise *Physica Sacra* that hops had a preservative quality which kept beer from spoiling after a couple of days. That allowed for a commercialization beyond anything gruit could offer, spawning a "hop tax" as well as condemnations from teetotalers for being a "wicked and pernicious weed."

If these things seem oddly familiar in the Age of Cannabis legalization, there is good reason. Hops (*humulus lupulus*) are botanical cousins of the beloved but oft misunderstood *cannabis* plants. And like pot, the green flower buds of the female hop plants are the most potent part. As far as beer brewing goes, the active ingredients in hops are acids and essential oils, which give them (and the beer) unique flavors and aromas. Like pot, different hops strains have different qualities. Those higher in alpha acids are good bittering agents, while others heavy on the beta acids are more aromatic, with scents often described as grassy, floral, citrus, spicy, piney, lemony, grapefruit and just plain earthy.

More to the point of our discussion, and theme of this book, hops are perhaps the healthiest ingredient in beer, having both antioxidant and antimicrobial properties. This should come as no surprise because they are green, and just about any green food you can name, from avocados to zucchini, is so healthy it probably has been proclaimed a "superfood" by one nutritionist or another. (We will discuss why you should eat more green food -- not including moldy bread or green beer on St. Patrick's Day -- later on.)

Besides their preservative qualities, the key to hops' health benefits is the antioxidant xanthohumol, a hard-to-spell flavonoid with antiviral, anti-inflammatory, anti-clotting, anti-tumor and anti-anxiety properties. All of those antis are a plus for whatever ails you as well as the dietary supplement industry, which offers numerous varieties of hop-derived elixirs. Unfortunately, there is such a miniscule amount of xanthohumol in beer you would have to drink massive quantities to reap substantial benefits, and the negative effects of our old nemesis alcohol would surely outweigh the good.

However, beer in general is a rich source of polyphenols, a class of antioxidants that help fight inflammatory ailments (which includes most types of chronic diseases), according to a 2016 review published in the journal *Nutrition, Metabolism and Cardiovascular Disease*.

Hops also have estrogen-mimicking compounds, which may benefit post-menopausal women. In fact, a study was done on a hoppy vaginal gel, but despite my affection for both vaginas and hops, I really don't want to go there.

To sum up: Hops add taste and aroma to beer, help to preserve it and contain some awesome antioxidants but ultimately don't have a lot of impact on beer bellies.

Yeast: The single-cell fungi collectively called yeast is the final ingredient in beer, both on this list and in the brewing process. While the malt and hops need to be boiled to catalyze the beer-making chemical reactions, yeast can't stand the heat. So you have to wait until the end of the boil, then cool the malt and hops concoction (called wort) to a temperate seventy-five degrees or so before adding the yeast. That's for ale yeast, as opposed to lager yeast, which likes things even cooler. In either case, if the yeast is happy, it will start eating the fermentable sugars, pooping out both carbon dioxide gas and alcohol. This turns your fermenter into a bubbling cauldron for a couple of days until the engorged, sated yeast settles in a dormant state on the bottom like your engorged great uncle Jack may settle on the sofa in a dormant state after Thanksgiving dinner (lager yeast actually ferments on the bottom, but that's kind of beside the point).

The yeast that fermented ancient beer was wild, coming from the air or where it had nestled in the cracks of the vessels that stored grain. Although early brewers had no idea what the yeast was, they did have the good sense to realize that it could turn barley grain-water into a drink with euphoric, even aphrodisiacal, qualities. They also learned that they could save some of the yeast sludge from the last batch to use in the next one. It all must have seemed magical since no one really knew exactly what the fermentation process involved, just that it happened. A gift from God.

In the mid-1800s, the famed French scientist Louis Pasteur finally figured it out how God did it. He also discovered bacteria in beer and a process to eradicate it, now called pasteurization. Today, this process is most closely associated with milk. But Pasteur was actually trying to figure out how to keep beer from going bad. So you can thank beer for pasteurized milk.

Along with CO2 and alcohol, yeast creates other byproducts that can flavor beer, primarily fruity esters and spicy phenols. Meanwhile, brewer's yeast taken as a supplement provides a lot of nutrients. But since you only ingest small amounts of yeast in a finished beer (especially in the filtered, pasteurized commercial varieties) these nutrients have limited impact and are thus not particularly relevant to our discussion. What is more relevant is that yeast transforms sugar into alcohol, which is not only calorie-dense but also metabolizes in a way that can compound weight gain, something we will look at in more detail when we get around to our chapter on alcohol.

To sum up: The small amount of yeast you consume in beer has a little nutritional impact, but one of its byproducts - alcohol - is loaded with calories that could contribute to a beer belly.

Beer Break

It's Friday afternoon and I've just cracked open a 22-ounce "bomber" bottle of Quadraphonic, a 10.5 percent ABV Belgian-style quadrupel ale from Barrel of Monks, my favorite local brewery in Boca Raton, Florida. The dark amber fluid cradles a cornucopia of aromas and flavors that tickle the nose and pleasure the palate. I not only savor the taste of this Belgian delight, but also the buzz. It packs a wallop but enhances without overwhelming. I feel relaxed, yet energized. My mind wanders freely, exploring the nooks and crannies of my creativity. Other inebriants may just numb you out. Quadraphonic pokes you in the ribs with a wink and says: "Watch this!"

So what makes Quadraphonic so special?

For one thing, it's hand-crafted with love. The brewery was founded by a pair of radiologists who seem more interested in making good beer than money. They say it took them a long time to develop Quadraphonic, and they continue to tinker with the recipe to perfect it. But it tastes just right to me. It lacks the bitter hop flavor you find in pale ales and IPAs, but that allows its incredibly complex malt profile to shine through strong. It's accented by an estery Belgian yeast, which adds undertones of dark fruit, such as figs, raisins and plums. All of these things blend together seamlessly, like a work of liquid art. Quadraphonic is a beer to be cherished, not gulped down on a hot day or chugged by an upside-down rugby player. Each sip needs to be appreciated, because you only have so many sips before the bottle is empty and, at 10.5 percent ABV, you can't have more lest the demon alcohol ambush you. There's a fine line between dancing with the Demon and being incapacitated by him, a line every beer-drinker should at least be aware of before deciding to back off or forge ahead, despite the consequences.

The Truth About Beer Bellies

Getting back to our discussion, I hope I didn't bore you by explaining how the primary ingredients in beer may contribute to your current or potential beer belly. But I'm sure you'll soon be delighted to finally hear why experts are probably right in declaring that beer belly-like gut protuberances are not really due to beer. They are much more about total calories consumed along with genetics, age and gender. The calories in beer do not promote a beer gut any more than the calories in wine, whiskey or French fries. In fact, now that you know what's in beer, you can see that there's very little outside of the alcohol and a few carbs from the malt that will contribute to any kind of weight gain, including beer bellies.

Basically, when you take in more calories than you burn up, it gets stored as fat. The body generally doesn't create more fat cells to store the excess but just makes the existing ones bigger. Depending on the rest of your physicality, the fat will accumulate faster or slower, and in different places. Some people who drink a lot of beer remain thin, while others who drink no beer at all can, ironically, develop beer bellies.

In this regard, women are kind of lucky. Most likely, it's because their bellies are reserved for more important things than fat - namely babies - so Mother Nature designed them to primarily store their excess calories as subcutaneous fat, the layer just under the skin. This type of fat tends to accumulate in the hips, butt, thighs and upper arms.

Whereas cottage cheese thighs and bat wings are not particularly attractive, they are fairly harmless compared to what men are more likely to develop: visceral fat in the gut. Among other unpleasantries, visceral fat is a marker of metabolic syndrome, a collection of symptoms that dramatically raises risk for diabetes, heart disease and stroke. Visceral fat also inhibits the fat-regulating hormone adiponectin, crippling a key soldier in your battle of the bulge. Furthermore, it triggers systemic inflammation, which promotes a host of chronic ailments. And visceral fat can actually squeeze your internal organs until they stop functioning properly.

Even skinny people can have deposits of visceral fat, but usually it manifests itself in waist circumference. As a rule of thumb (or perhaps gut) men should maintain a waist-size under forty inches, and for women the magic number is thirty-five. That is one reason why I'm always crowing about being in my sixties, drinking lots of beer and still fitting into size 32 trousers.

While the beer belly may be a myth, there's little doubt that drinking too much beer can exacerbate a weight problem for a few reasons. The first is that beer is liquid calories, which are not as filling as solid food calories. A 12-ounce bottle of beer can have upwards of two hundred calories, which isn't as likely to fill you up as much as the two hundred calories you get when you eat two bananas or apples, or even a beef patty.

Another reason is that alcohol increases appetite, at least in lab mice. There's been no definitive study done on humans, but British researchers found that alcohol stimulated AgRP neurons in the hypothalamus of the rodents' brains, which gave them a serious case of the munchies. The scientists figure the same holds true for people, something any bartender will confirm. Alcohol is also a diuretic, meaning we piss it away, which lowers our body's levels of electrolytes, including sodium. So we not only get hungry when we booze it up but also start craving salty foods such as nachos, mozzarella sticks, chicken wings and other barroom staples. The perfect fat storm is completed by our alcohol-induced loss of inhibitions, prompting us to say fuhgeddabout the sensible house salad and go with the bacon-cheeseburger and onion rings.

So while we all should be relieved to know that the beer belly is a myth, you can't expect to indulge in beer and bar food, and still maintain a slim waistline. On the other hand, I manage to drink more beer than the AMA recommends, lose inhibitions and pig out on bar food at times and, need I say it, still fit into size 32 pants. Read on to learn how I do it, and how you can, too!

Chapter 3
Taking Responsibility for Drinking Irresponsibly

How much beer do you drink? Really.

It's a question beer-lovers don't like to hear. We don't want to count, or be held accountable. We just want to enjoy the epicurean delights and warm, fuzzy feelings our brews bestow on us in peace and harmony. Still, deep down we know that our body counts each one, and it will eventually hold us accountable.

I'd say I average about three beers a day, or 50 percent over the AMA's recommended guidelines for men. Not too bad, until you consider those three beers are higher in alcohol and calories than your average brew. Three of mine are probably equal to four Budweisers. So now I'm up to double the AMA's red line, which suddenly seems like a lot.

It *is* a lot. More than sensible. The problem is that beer makes me nonsensible, and I drink more than I should. While the easiest way to enjoy beer and not have it expand the waistline and damage health is to drink responsibly, it is hardly something that I, and many beer-lovers, can consistently do. We have a tendency to overindulge, because we simply love beer. Even when we try to drink it slowly and savor every sip, it is still gone too soon. That can lead to another, and another, which puts us over the AMA's threshold for a safe daily intake. It's a bit of a quandary. Besides consuming all of those the liquid calories, when you cross that red line of two beers a day for a man and one for a woman, the AMA, sobriety organizations and a vast number of researchers warn that you are increasing risk for an assortment of ailments, including heart and liver disease, various types of cancer, mental problems, sexual dysfunction and memory loss, the latter of which can cause you to more often forget where you left your beer after you put it down somewhere to attend to something other than drinking it.

Of course, there are also plenty of us who can push the envelope and not wind up with things like heart disease and cancer, and for whom beer seems to enhance mental health and sexual function. The problem is most of us don't always know where we are on the scale. One option is not worry about it and drink up until one day you experience pain or dysfunction somewhere in your body, go to the doctor and find out that your days, and beers, are numbered. A better option is to take responsibility for your own health now and be proactive in trying to lessen the impact of excessive beer consumption.

On a couple of occasions, I've interviewed neurologist Dr. James Galvin, founding director of the Center for Comprehensive Brain Health at Florida Atlantic University in Boca Raton. While we didn't discuss beer (I'm sure he'd strongly recommend complying with the AMA guidelines), much of what he said about his specialty, dementia, relates to our topic because what's good for the brain is good for the beer-drinker. When asked what the best thing a person can do to lower risk of developing Alzheimer's and other neurodegenerative conditions, Galvin planted his tongue firmly in cheek and replied: "Pick your parents well."

"Even though many diseases aren't genetic, your gene pool plays a role," he explained. "You also learn a lot of your behaviors from your parents, so if they have unhealthy habits, you're more likely to have them too."

Of course, we don't pick our parents any more than they pick us. We just kind of end up with each other. But we can see reflections of ourselves in them, including many of our strengths and weaknesses.

As I write this, my mother is ninety-three years old, still lives on her own, drives a car, serves as a docent at an art museum and can read her morning newspaper without glasses. She's able to do all of this despite never having formally exercised a day in her life, at least not since I've known her, which is sixty-six years (not counting *in utero*). She does eat pretty well, drinks well within the AMA guidelines, and exercises her brain by studying up on all of the new art museum exhibits, reading a lot of books, doing the *New York Times* crossword puzzle and favoring PBS over less cerebral TV options.

My dad, on the other hand, suffered the first of his three heart attacks at age forty-three, and died at seventy-two after a bout with stomach and liver cancer. But what my father lacked in longevity genes, he made up for in attitude. Although he had what should have been debilitating heart problems, he lived life to the fullest, traveling, skiing, swimming, boating, drinking an occasional scotch, running a factory and pretty much making everyone around him happy and joyful and not scared of life. He always used to say he was "psychosomatically well." So it's a mixed bag for me. Since I haven't had any genetic testing, I really don't know exactly what I've inherited. So far, it looks like I got my mom's healthy aging and my dad's psychosomatic wellness, but I should also watch out for heart disease and cancer.

While it's good to be aware of your health heritage, that's not something you can control any more than you can pick your parents.

So what can you do to be proactive about your health in order to better tolerate more beer than the AMA's average man or woman?

Well, that largely depends on you. And that brings us back to Dr. Galvin. He's fond of saying, "A one-size-fits-all approach fits no one." We are all different; our needs are different; and we react to things differently, including beer. Galvin runs the Dementia Prevention Program, which consists of extensive diagnostic testing - brain scans, blood panels, cognitive tests, sleep studies, lifestyle evaluations and a psychological profile - to determine dementia risk factors, such as obesity, type 2 diabetes, hypertension, depression, sleep apnea and rugby. Then he and his team devise a personal program for each patient to reduce the risks. You might need nutritional supplements or medications, or changes in diet or lifestyle, or retiring from rugby after getting your bell rung too many times.

In similar fashion, you can do a less formal beer capacity diagnosis of your own by looking at your family history, health history, blood work and weekly beer tab. Then you can make adjustments to optimize your health, because a healthy body will not only stave off the onset of dementia but also tolerate the stress of beer overconsumption better than an unhealthy body. Obviously, if one or both of your parents suffered from alcoholism, you need to realize you are much more likely to suffer from it too.

The key is to take responsibility for your own health. Don't wait until something hurts to go to a doctor. Don't let the doctor just dictate what you should do. Find a physician who will work with you to keep you healthy rather than just prescribe drugs when something goes wrong. Learn about health and aging. A lot of people know more about how their car works than their bodies. Learn how your body works. If you're diagnosed with a medical problem, study up about it in books, on websites or even YouTube, so you can knowledgeably work with a doctor or some other healer rather than just blindly putting yourself in their hands. Get in touch with your body through exercise, stretching, meditation, yoga, sex, self-exams, mirror-gazing and anything else that helps you to understand the norm so you can quickly recognize when something goes amiss. The sooner you catch a problem, the easier you can deal with it.

This is a very important lesson: Take responsibility for your health to help reduce the impact of being irresponsible about how much beer you may drink.

Chapter 4
A Question of Balance

What makes a great beer?

I ponder this question on the last Sunday of the year, after a morning bike ride to Deerfield Beach under sunny skies with the temperature hovering around seventy-five degrees. The sub-tropics are nice this time of year; not too hot, not too cold. None of the early afternoon pro football games matter at this point in the season, so I steal some time to sit and think and write and drink beer.

I have before me a glass of Winter Storm, an Imperial ESB (Extra Special Bitter) produced by the Heavy Seas brewery in Maryland. As the name implies, it's a winter beer, ironically my favorite season for brews often called "warmers," even though I live in a place that rarely chills the bones. I always enjoy Winter Storm during the few months it's around, along with Santa's Reserve from Rogue brewery in Oregon, and a British series from Ridgeway named for some of Santa's more twisted helpers (Bad Elf, Very Bad Elf, Seriously Bad Elf, Criminally Bad Elf and Insanely Bad Elf). Winter Storm is a dark ruby ale with frothy but fleeting head that blends bitter West Coast Warrior hops, earthy Goldings and Fuggle aromatic hops from Britain, malts with sweet caramel and chocolate undertones, and a substantial but not overwhelming 7.5 percent ABV.

Ultimately, what makes Winter Storm so special is balance. All of the parts may pull and tug on each other, but they come together in the end to produce a beer that is bitter, but not too bitter; sweet, but not too sweet; and boozy, but not too boozy.

It's good to be well-balanced, whether you're a beer or a human. Your body works best when it is in balance physically, emotionally and chemically. Fortunately, our bodies strive to keep us that way, a process known as homeostasis. For example, when our blood sugar spikes from downing a bottle of Brooklyn Black Chocolate Stout (10 percent ABV, 320 calories), our pancreas secretes more insulin to help process the rush of sugars.

But if we challenge our body too much, it can't keep up and loses its balance. In the case of blood sugar, the insulin loses effectiveness. Basically, our cells get so saturated with sugar the insulin can't transport any more of it through the cell membranes, so it just stays in the blood. This is called insulin resistance and can eventually lead to type 2 diabetes. If you have type 2 diabetes, chances are your doctor will order you to cut down or eliminate your consumption of Brooklyn Black Chocolate Stout, and probably any other beers that don't have "lite" or "ultra" in their names. That, in turn, will get your spouse, kids and/or parents to pester you about your beer consumption, so you begin to feel guilty and lose some of the vast pleasures of imbibing. The complications associated with type 2 diabetes, which include heart disease, blindness, nerve pain and amputation, can also damper your beer-drinking pleasures.

The good news is that drinking a few, or even several, Brooklyn Black Chocolate Stouts won't in itself cause type 2 diabetes. But if you combine it with the typical high-sugar, high-carb, processed food diet of many if not most Americans, it will definitely increase the risk of having something else for your mother to nag you about.

Drinking too much beer can throw other bodily systems out of balance, including your whole body, such as in, "I've fallen and I can't get up!" But it really pesters the liver, which has more than five hundred functions but has to put a lot of stuff on the back burner to process the poison alcohol and get it through the system and out of the body as quickly as possible. Eventually, the liver can get permanently damaged, and you can die, which will definitely put a crimp in your beer drinking pleasures.

Beer Fast

But there's more good news. The liver is regenerative (like a salamander's tail) and can repair itself if given a break and the damage isn't too severe. I can thank my mother for helping me to give myself such a break every year. Back in the early 1980s, I was crashing at my parents' oceanfront condo in Fort Lauderdale while penning a novel about my nearly two years of backpacking vagabondage around Europe and the Middle East. Along with writing, I was playing rugby with the Fort Lauderdale Knights and drinking quantities of beer that your average rugby player would consider moderate, but excessive by most other people's standards, including my mother. She was convinced I was becoming an alcoholic and bet me a nickel (her standard wager) that I could not quit drinking for a month. I accepted the bet and picked February 17 to March 17 because a) February is the shortest month, and b) I could break my beer fast on St. Patrick's Day, arguably the best drinking day of the year. Since that timeframe roughly coincides with the forty days Catholics deprive themselves of various pleasures, my mother dubbed it "Jewish Lent." I did it then, and I have done it ever since.

Although a pain in the ass, not drinking alcohol for an extended period of time is interesting. It really changes your perspective when you go out partying with pals and/or loved ones. They are bright-eyed, alert and square-shouldered at the start, but devolve as the night progresses. Their eyelids start to droop and shoulders sag, as though gravity has more of a tug on them with each downed beer. You don't notice it as much when you're drinking along with them. But now they seem sillier and dumber than normal, and their breath smells like a frat house on Sunday morning. They're also more likely to share overly warm and fuzzy feelings with you until they finally pay their tab and Uber off into the night. It's hard to believe the same thing happens to you, to some degree, for the rest of the year. But it also plants a seed deep in your unconscious that, in the future, will sometimes stay your hand before downing a beer you don't really need.

At some point, I shifted my beer fast to January. Even though it is tied for the longest month, there's not much on my social drinking calendar in January, whereas February has the Fort Lauderdale Ruggerfest and a local Renaissance festival, which are both very challenging to enjoy without beer. Since I start my beer fast on the day after New Year's Day (no sense stopping in the middle of the night, especially with a full lineup of the top college football games on TV later in the day), I now break it on Groundhog Day. Like a movie of the same name, it involves a recurring activity - pour, drink, repeat - until my eyelids start to droop and shoulders sag.

Coincidentally, a Britain-based nonprofit called Alcohol Research UK began promoting a "Dry January" in 2013, and five years later more than three million Brits pledged to basically follow what I've been doing for decades. And at least one scientific study showed that the month's abstinence from alcohol not only improved liver function but also lowered blood sugar levels and resulted in weight loss. So it would seem that, physiologically, going a month without beer and other alcoholic beverages helps to at least partially balance out the effects of indulging during the rest of the year.

It really sucks to not drink any beer (or wine, or whiskey, or even sake) for a whole month, but I'm still doing it. I'm doing something good for my health, and I'm making my mom happy (I never did collect on that nickel bet). I also lose five to ten pounds for a while and save a couple hundred bucks that otherwise would have been spent on beer. A little sacrifice goes a long way for these reasons and more. Truth is, to fully appreciate anything, you have to deny yourself of it from time to time.

In other words, abstinence makes the heart grow fonder.

Chapter 5
Starving Writer

Homo sapiens have been around for about 300,000 years, and for all but a tiny fraction of that time, our primary occupation was the procurement of food. To provide nourishment, animals were hunted down and edible vegetation was gathered up. It was a full-time job just to amass enough food to survive. Nowadays, it's as easy as driving on over to the local supermarket. Although finding a parking spot in the supermarket lot can be challenging, and even confrontational, it's a lot less challenging and confrontational then, say, killing and butchering a wooly mammoth, as some of our ancient ancestors used to do.

In many ways, we have come a long way since then (much farther, in fact, than the wooly mammoth), but the evolution of our bodies hasn't really changed much since the days of cavemen and cavewomen, who sometimes had to go days, or even weeks, between meals. They survived because their bodies had evolved to be incredibly efficient in how energy was used and stored. Not a calorie of wooly mammoth meat nor any other food went unused for long. What the body needed for immediate energy was burned, and anything remaining after a day was converted to fat and stored until it was tapped for energy when food was scarce.

Since food was so often scarce, fat was regularly burned off and didn't have a chance to accumulate. Although it's impossible to tell from fossilized bones, there probably weren't any chubby cavemen like Jack Black in the movie *Year One,* nor bombshell cavewomen busting out of their furry bikinis like Raquel Welch in *One Million Years B.C.* They burned massive amounts of calories just to survive, trekking through rugged terrain, hunting down animals, hauling water, climbing trees and even shivering to keep warm.

World of Excess

Cut to the 21st century, the Age of Uber Eats, where we don't have to get off of our butts to procure food. With climate-controlled living quarters, we don't even shiver much these days. And, oh, what a wondrous assortment of nourishment we have. The average supermarket stocks some 40,000 items, mostly food. That's more than five times what they had when I was growing up in the 1960s. Never before in the history of humankind have we had such a vast selection of food from around the globe, and it's all available for purchase at the neighborhood supermarket or specialty store.

It's not only easy to gather this sustenance, but thanks to shopping carts, we don't even have to carry it around, except maybe from car to kitchen. And it's easily affordable, costing us, on average, less than 6 percent of our household income. Spend a little more, and we can have experts prepare the food for our consumption at countless restaurants offering the full spectrum of Planet Earth's cuisines. We can even find several different cuisines in the same place, like the Bacchanal Buffet at Caesar's Palace, which offers an all-you-can-eat buffet featuring more than five hundred dishes…French soufflés, American barbecue, Japanese sushi...geez, I'm getting hungry just writing about this stuff.

We live in a culinary nirvana, a Garden of Eating where all of the fruit is low hanging. It's easily plucked, prepped and popped into the mouth to please the palate and sate the tummy, fulfilling a primordial urge to feast before the inevitable famine.

But the famine is no longer inevitable, or even likely here in the good old USA. That creates a dilemma because we weren't designed to be able to eat all we want whenever we want, and adding beer's liquid calories to the equation exacerbates the problem. So we need some form of self-restraint. This is why diets were developed. They were also developed to make money and have become a multibillion-dollar industry despite the troubling fact that diets generally don't work. Most dieters – some studies estimate upwards of 90 percent – may drop a few pounds initially but gain it all back, and often more, within five years.

So how have I managed to lose most of my mid-life weight gain and not put it back on for more than a decade despite consistently drinking a lot of high-calorie craft beer and homebrew?

Well, for one thing, I don't diet. And I'm not exactly a bastion of self-restraint. Actually, it all goes back to my son Glen's asthma. He was diagnosed with the breathing disorder as an infant and suffered a couple or three severe attacks a year. He'd start coughing, usually at night, and not stop for days despite treatment with things like steroids, inhalants, antibiotics and heavy doses of Cartoon Network.

When Glen was in fifth grade, he suffered an asthma attack that wouldn't abate. After his pediatrician and pediatric pulmonary specialist failed to suppress it with drugs, including a potent codeine cough syrup, my wife Nora and I took him to see Dr. Corey Cameron. She's a chiropractor and holistic healer who'd helped a friend of ours beat a mysterious lupus-like condition she'd been battling for years.

Tall, attractive and self-assured, Dr. Corey reminded me of Mary Poppins, floating into our lives to make everything better, seemingly by magic -- but definitely without the spoonful of sugar and medicine. She examined Glen by not only doing a standard chiropractic resistance test to identify trouble spots in the spine, but also a version to identify underperforming internal organs. After giving Glen a once-over, Dr. Corey declared that the problem had nothing to do with his lungs but rather his heart. She explained that its life force energy was low, and the brain, in an effort to stimulate the heart, was triggering the cough reflex. That seemed a stretch to me, but after Dr. Corey treated Glen with a spinal adjustment, heart-specific nutrients, essential oils and some kind of light therapy, his cough subsided for the most part and was gone by the time he went to sleep that night.

If you're beginning to wonder what all of this has to do about drinking beer without piling on pounds, hold on as I'm getting around to discussing how Dr. Corey introduced me to what I consider to be the single most effective thing I do to combat weight gain. But I'd like to take a moment to stress that healing comes in many forms, some of which may seem bizarre to those of us raised primarily with care through conventional medical doctors, who typically treat ailments with an assortment of drugs and procedures. We tend to seek their help after something goes wrong, hoping they can fix it. Often they can, at least temporarily. They happen to be very good at fixing us when we break ourselves in car wrecks and rugby games, but their track record in battling disease is mixed, at best.

Dr. Galvin, who you'll recall runs the Dementia Prevention Program (if you're not already suffering from dementia), once told me: "I'm going to let you in on a secret. Doctors can't cure disease, with the exception of most bacterial infections and some cancers. Everything else we just treat. We can't cure diabetes, arthritis, hypertension, multiple sclerosis, Alzheimer's or any other chronic disease, but we can prevent them. And if you don't develop a disease, there's no need to cure it."

In recent decades, more and more emphasis has been put on preventative care, something that has long been the focus of chiropractors, acupuncturists, aromatherapists, Chinese herbalists and other alternative medicine practitioners. A new breed of MDs has emerged, those who practice functional or integrative medicine. They embrace both mainstream and alternative methods, but typically consider drugs and surgeries to be last resorts rather than first options. Some of them have been ostracized by the stodgy AMA, but they never-the-less are growing in numbers and popularity.

The bottom line is that you shouldn't be afraid to explore alternative care, especially if the conventional docs aren't helping whatever ails you. After seeing Dr. Corey, Glen continued to have an occasional asthma attack, but they never approached the severity he experienced before seeing her. As I write this, he's now twenty-five and hasn't had so much as a wheeze in many years.

Dr. Corey also wound up treating Nora, who was soon able to shuck the prescription medications she'd been taking for asthma, arthritis, vertigo and depression. When Glen started coughing again a couple of months after his initial visit to Dr. Corey, I whisked him back to her office. While I went to work, Dr. Corey and her staff of two kept Glen all afternoon, treating him with nutrients, "lights," TLC and even a tuna fish sandwich. By the time I arrived to pick him up, he was no longer coughing. But as we were waiting by the counter to settle our bill, he started up again, and it got worse as the evening progressed. So the next day I brought him back to Dr. Corey, who examined him and proclaimed that he was fine, even as he continued to cough every few seconds. She looked at me, her eyes narrowing.

"I think it's you," she said, and performed some of her seemingly mumbo-jumbo diagnostic tests on me.

"It is," she concluded. "You're a sucker."

"I guess I am," I thought, *"because now I'm going to end up paying to have you treat me even though my health is fine."*

Dr. Corey explained that sometimes people with weaknesses drain strength from those who are close to them, and she believed that was the case with Glen and me. She adjusted my spine and gave me some nutrients to boost my heart energy. Incredibly, Glen stopped coughing as soon as I popped the pills in my mouth. If you find this hard to believe, you are not alone. I still find it hard to believe, even though it happened to me. But as Dr. Corey is fond of saying, "The proof is in the pudding." And thus she managed to rope the whole family into her alternative care.

Intermittent Fasting

While seeing Dr. Corey, our whole family's health improved. But I was also reaching my zenith as far as weight goes. Coincidentally, Dr. Corey had a patient whose health took a dramatic turn for the better after she started using products and following a protocol developed by a dietary supplement company called Isagenix. It was a two-prong approach that consisted of combining good nutrition with a regular cleansing fast. Nora and I tried it, starting with their 9-Day Cleanse, which consisted of a two-day cleansing fast with no food, followed by five days of subsisting on two high-quality undenatured whey protein shakes and one small meal a day, followed by another two-day cleansing fast. It was no fun, but by the end we had each dropped several pounds and felt great. I still do one 9-Day Cleanse a year, right at the end of my January beer fast. More importantly, I do a cleansing fast once a week, usually on Monday, because Mondays generally suck anyway.

I later learned that what I do is called intermittent fasting, which is denying your body of sustenance for a specific period of time. It's what our cavemen ancestors did out of necessity rather than choice. There are a few different varieties of intermittent fasting, but they all work on the same principles. When you don't eat for several hours, your body starts depleting its blood glucose fuel supply and burning fat instead. It also redirects the energy needed for digestion over to the body's repair and maintenance department. Those two things trigger a bunch of healthy physiological changes. I don't want to bore you with the details of the very complex biochemical processes involved (in part because I would have to look them all up), but scientific studies show that intermittent fasting improves insulin sensitivity to help fight diabetes, decreases fat mass, lowers blood pressure, reduces the kind of systemic inflammation associated with most chronic diseases, reduces oxidative stress that damages cells and DNA, promotes brain health, and facilitates a process called autophagy, which is how dysfunctional cells break themselves down and recycle their parts to form new, healthy cells.

In other words, it's all good.

Dr. Jason Fung, a Canadian kidney specialist, once explained to me that one sure way to beat diabetes is to stop eating, at least temporarily. He was interested in diabetes because the disease damages kidneys. While that may have been good for his business, it was bad for his diabetic patients, many of whom ended up on dialysis. Fung conducted a small but significant study on insulin-dependent diabetics, who not only needed injections of the hormone that processes glucose to keep their blood sugar levels under control, but also other prescription medications. The good doctor put them on an intermittent fasting regimen that consisted of them not eating for twenty-four hours every other day.

"On fasting days, they skipped breakfast and lunch, basically going from dinner to dinner without eating," says Fung, author of *The Complete Guide to*

Fasting. "They had no trouble complying, and we saw incredible results almost right away. All of them were off insulin in five to eighteen days, and they'd been on it for years. Their blood sugar is better now than when they were on insulin and medications, which means the underlying disease is better."

There are several other intermittent fasting protocols, with the most popular being the 16/8 and 5/2 plans. In the first, you eat whatever you want, but all within an eight-hour window, such as 10 a.m. to 6 p.m. So you fast sixteen hours a day. In the second, you eat normally five days a week and either fast completely or eat just 500-600 calories on the other two days.

As for me, I eat nothing from Sunday night until Tuesday morning, which is about thirty-four hours. I do drink four ounces of Isagenix's Cleanse for Life solution mixed with a big glass of water, four times during that period. Cleanse for Life is a proprietary blend including extracts of alfalfa leaf, burdock root, aloe vera leaf, licorice root, bilberry, pau d'arco bark, fennel seed, turmeric root, rhodiola root and a lot of other roots, barks and herbs that have been used for health in traditional medicine throughout the ages. According to the folks at Isagenix, the concoction helps induce cells to release toxins so they can be eliminated by the body. Since toxins are mostly stored in fat cells, getting rid of them will shrink the fat cells. So, one of the side effects of removing toxins is weight loss.

The morning after my fast, I feel a bit drained. But as soon as I start fueling up with the whey protein shake and other food, my energy levels skyrocket, and I soon feel as though I can walk through walls. That feeling lasts two or three days, until the beer and, eventually, weekend festivities drag me back down to earth. By Monday, I'm craving my cleansing fast, even though actually doing it is somewhat torturous. The hunger itself isn't so bad. I mostly miss the ritual of breaking bread with loved ones (or even the newspaper) and the corporeal pleasures of eating, which rival the pleasures of sex. We were designed to crave food, and those cravings are much more powerful than whatever discomfort we may physically feel from an empty belly. On the plus side, I don't have to wash any dishes that day.

I have fasted without Cleanse for Life on occasion, just drinking purified water, but don't seem to get the same kick. There are a lot of cleansing drinks you can try, including things like lemon water and green tea. The internet offers a variety of homemade cleansing drink recipes, and there are dozens of other cleansing concoctions produced by other companies.

In any case, the best thing about my weekly food sacrifice is it's like hitting a reset button that gives my body a fresh start. I may shift the fast to other days, usually Tuesday if Monday is a holiday, but rarely miss a week. I've been doing it for about a decade now, and I credit it for being a major reason why I can drink a lot of beer and not gain weight.

Beerless Break

All this talk about not eating, or drinking beer, is getting me depressed, as I often am on Mondays with little to look forward to except finally getting through the day and evening and going to sleep so I can wake up and eat again. While I can't actually take a beer break today, a little mental beer break may help. I spin the wheel of fond beer memories…

…and it lands in the early years of the new millennium, when I discovered a whole New World of Beer in a small shop in the northeast corner of a nondescript strip mall.

I was freelance writing, and my primary client was American Media, Inc. (AMI), publishers of the supermarket tabloids National Enquirer, Globe, Star and others, including my favorite, the late, great Weekly World News, in which my son Glen once appeared as the Kangaroo Kid, a plucky Australian boy who'd tragically lost his legs in an accident but had a double kangaroo leg transplant and proudly declared, "I'm the only kid in my class who can slam dunk a basketball."

I'd typically work at AMI's Boca Raton headquarters a few days a week, churning out gossipy stories about celebrities and special sections like "Scandals of the Beauty Queens" or "America's Natural Born Killers." About a month after the 9/11 terrorist attacks rocked our world, AMI suffered an anthrax attack that killed photo editor Bob Stevens, sickened a few others who survived, and forced us out of the contaminated building. We landed in a dark, cramped temporary office we called The Bunker. The walls were painted black, there were no windows, and the desks were lined up with no space between them.

Although The Bunker was not far from the anthrax building, I took a different route home and passed by a small bottle shop called Case & Keg, but had big letters on the side of the building spelling out WORLD OF BEER. I'd seen the place before but had never stopped. Publix had a pretty good selection of imported beer at decent prices, and at that point I figured Beck's and Carlsberg were about as good as it got.

But one day on my way home from The Bunker, I stopped in the Case & Keg and was delighted to find that they carried Whitbread, Tartan Bitter and some other beers

I'd encountered overseas but were hard to come by in the States. I bought a couple of six-packs, and returned the next week, and week after that, and so on, for more.

The managing partner, Jeff, eventually pointed out some American beers he said I should try. They were from so-called microbreweries scattered about the country. Since Jeff seemed to know a lot more about beer than I did, I followed his advice. While knowing that choosing a beer by its bottle is like choosing a book by its cover, I still went with Rogue's Dead Guy Ale because I liked the name and label, which had a skeleton with mug in hand sitting on a wooden cask. Jeff approved, and it turned out to be as good, or better, than my beloved imports.

I made a habit of going to the Case & Keg once a week, usually on Fridays when they had tastings, and coming home with a different beer each time. Once, the guy from Shmaltz Brewing was there, carting around cases of He'Brew Genesis – "The Chosen Beer" – in an old Volvo. I tried a sample of the amber ale and was sold. Shmaltz no longer makes Genesis but has consistently good stuff, my favorite being Bittersweet Lenny's R.I.P.A., a 10 percent ABV rye double IPA with "an obscene amount of malt and hops" dedicated to shock comedy legend Lenny Bruce.

One December, Jeff pointed out a special holiday release he'd just gotten in. Like Dead Guy Ale, it was from Rogue brewery in Oregon, but called Santa's Reserve. I passed on it due to its exorbitant $12.99 price tag, then changed my mind a few days later and went back. He was already sold out, and I had to wait a whole year to finally try it. But it was worth the wait, and I haven't missed it since.

I got to be such a regular customer that Jeff used to let me stash a hundred pounds of live crawfish -- flown in from New Orleans -- in his cooler overnight before Nora's annual crawfish boil birthday party (otherwise we'd have to put them on ice in the bathtub, which got messy). Meanwhile, I could go on and on about all of the beers I discovered at Case & Keg, which boasted of having the largest selection in Florida.

Then Total Wine opened up a few miles away. The selection there was bigger and the prices lower. I continued to patronize Case & Keg out of loyalty, until the stock began to dwindle due to distribution demands Jeff could no longer meet. Before long, his once-thriving business fizzled out of existence, but it will always remain near and dear to my beer-loving heart.

More Good News

Okay. I feel a little better now. And it's closer to Tuesday, when I will eat, drink beer and be happy again. I recently came across some other good news about intermittent fasting. Because I do it, I might be less likely to ever get cancer, a disease so insidious and disturbing people used to not even utter the word and refer to in hushed tones as "The Big C." The reason why intermittent fasting may protect me against you-know-what is rather complicated and involves mitochondria, metabolic pathways, somatic mutations, the oncogenic paradox and other complex physiological things that would instantly send many beer-lovers into a coma-like stupor. Oddly enough, it also involves fermentation, but in a cellular metabolic manner that has absolutely nothing to do with beer.

A renegade researcher named Thomas Seyfried has rather convincing arguments and data to explain why we have been spinning our wheels in our seeming endless war against cancer. He says we've been fighting the wrong battle. While everyone thinks that cancer is driven by genetic mutations in cells, he is convinced that the root cause is metabolic, that is how cells process energy. The genetic defects that cause tumor growth, he says, are a downstream effect of the energy-generating dysfunction, and one of the ways to help right the metabolic ship is by fasting.

While interviewing Dr. Seyfried, a Boston College biology professor and author of *Cancer as a Metabolic Disease,* for an article about his revolutionary approach to fighting cancer - imagine treatment that is extremely effective, non-toxic and low-cost - I told him about my weekly cleansing fast.

"Well, you'll probably never have to worry about cancer," he said. "Of course, nothing is guaranteed, but therapeutic fasting is anti-angiogenic and pro-apoptotic, and thus targets multiple cancer hallmarks."

So that's another good reason to fast intermittently, because no one wants to be pro-angiogenic and anti-apoptotic, I guess, even if they don't know what that means.

Of course, the key to all of this good stuff is not eating even with a household full of lip-smacking foodstuffs and TV commercials constantly displaying succulent-looking meals from a variety of restaurants. Despite our ancient ancestors evolving in such a fashion that they could regularly go long periods without food, modern day humans can't seem to go more than a few hours without it, unless they're asleep. In fact, many people seem amazed that I can go all day without eating and claim they couldn't do it because they'd get headaches, heart palpitations or various other potentially crippling responses. But it's really not that hard, and you get used to it. As an added bonus, hunger has less of an impact on you even when you're not fasting, which translates into less impulse eating.

One reason intermittent fasting is so doable is that you know it is temporary. You never lose sight of the food (and beer) at the end of the tunnel, and it tastes better than ever when you finally get to eat it. To quote Cervantes: "Hunger is the best sauce." It is the temporary nature of intermittent fasting that makes it easier to comply with than diets, where you often are asked to give up certain things indefinitely. In contrast, intermittent fasting asks you to give up everything, but just for a limited time.

As far as Isagenix goes, it isn't the only company that produces these types of products. But I started with them and have always been satisfied, so I see no reason to try any of the others. Like a lot of nutritional supplement companies, Isagenix relies on network marketing, and their compensation program is reputed to be among the most generous in the industry. It certainly has been generous to Dr. Corey, who has become one of their top producers. In fact, she's made so much money from Isagenix she was able to retire from her practice. It's kind of sad in a way because she has a special gift that can help people like my son. But I'm sure she'd say she helps a lot more people by spreading the gospel of good health through Isagenix. Nora and I tried to get rich by network marketing the stuff, but our efforts never gelled. So I continue to write for a living. However, if you want to try Isagenix, we'd be happy to help you (email us at IsaGreenberg@gmail.com). That way, maybe we can develop a residual income stream to support our retirement.

But rest assured, no matter how much money I make, I will always be a starving writer, at least one day a week.

Chapter 6

What to Consume in Addition to Beer

When I was a kid, I didn't eat much of anything. I wouldn't touch pizza, pasta, rice, soup, regular milk, cheese, vegetables...hmmmm, I suppose it would be easier to list what I did eat: potato chips, pretzels, various cookies, cupcakes and donuts, candy (without nuts or coconut), ice cream (chocolate only), beef, fried flounder, potatoes in most forms, fried chicken, raw peas (only if they were still in their pods), applesauce, scrambled eggs, Nova lox (no bagel), and sandwiches made on white bread with butter and only bologna, kosher salami, bacon or tuna fish. I also ate peanut butter (creamy) and jelly (strawberry) on white bread with no butter. I didn't eat bread crusts but preferred them left on the bread rather than trimmed. I'd eat a hamburger patty or hot dog, but not on a bun, which I considered to be bread that was all crust. I washed it all down mainly with chocolate milk but also the full spectrum of sodas (except Mountain Dew) and most fruit juices. I also liked to eat ice and took a one-a-day multiple vitamin. That's it, seriously.

It's a miracle I managed to survive, and even flourish, on this diet. I was rarely sick and a natural athlete who was one of the first kids chosen in pick-up games of anything even though I was always the shortest, scrawniest kid in my class. I'm not sure how I managed to stay so functional while eating such a lousy diet and can only chalk it up to the incredible resiliency of the young human body. I remained a picky eater extremist into my college years at Penn State, when I slowly began to expand my culinary horizons to include pizza, spaghetti, Velveeta grilled cheese sandwiches and, finally, bread crusts. For the most part, I rejected all green food with the exception of iceberg lettuce slathered with one particular brand of creamy garlic dressing.

I did, however, make great strides in my major food group, sandwiches, after landing a job at the Stage Door Deli in downtown State College, Pennsylvania. I started out doing deliveries but eventually worked my way up to sandwich-maker. There were 110 different sandwiches, all named after movie stars. Roast beef varieties were Western stars, ham leading men, corn beef leading women, pastrami gangsters, liverwurst horror, and tuna aquatic female stars (insert politically incorrect joke here). People would order the sandwiches by the stars' names, such as a Clark Gable on rye (ham, coleslaw and Russian dressing), so we had to memorize them all.

By then I had swapped out the butter for mayonnaise on my sandwiches, and added exotic foods such as lettuce and tomato. Life went on and my tastes slowly expanded, then exploded when I traveled around Europe and the Middle East and often had to eat new foods or go hungry. Now, I eat pretty much anything, with notable exceptions being most olives and all cucumbers.

Oddly enough, when I started drinking beer, my tastes for it immediately broadened, as I found I liked the imported stuff much better than domestic varieties. And I was willing to pay for it. For example, in my favorite collegiate bar, Zeno's, I ordered 90-cent Heinekens instead of 75-cent Budweisers. Still, the choices back then were limited. My beer horizons expanded when I went overseas, first in Britain with pub brews such as Bass, Whitbread and especially Watney's bitter. Later in Germany, I was delighted to find that even small towns had their own breweries producing a variety of biers I'd never heard of before, and in most cases, since. But my first impression of German beer in Germany was crossing a bridge on my trusty Honda 250cc motorcycle into the city of Bremen and seeing a huge Beck's sign on the smokestacks of the brewery. I stopped at the first drinking establishment I saw, on a road right under the bridge, where a bartender drew me a Beck's draft in a stemmed glass with paper skirt. He leveled the frothy white head with a beer comb, then added another shot from the tap, again and again, slowly teasing the head until it extended inches over the rim of the glass…

Sorry. I do get carried away by fond memories of beer, and I really need to get around to the gist of this chapter, which is to enlighten you on the types of food that go best with beer if you don't want to get a pseudo beer belly.

So, my diet was pretty crappy most of my life, and I often subsisted on sandwiches piled high with cold cuts, a slice or two of cheese and maybe some lettuce and/or tomato that I could take or leave. I rarely ate a lunch that wasn't a sandwich, sometimes had one for dinner and, if out partying, a midnight snack.

Soup's On!

After encountering Dr. Corey and Isagenix, I began to take more of an interest in nutrition. I learned that eating upwards of two pounds of cold cuts a week probably wasn't in my best interest, since the heavily processed meat seems to have as many carcinogens as nutrients, not to mention fairly ridiculous levels of saturated fat and salt. Coincidentally, I chose a book called *Enlightened Soups*, by one Camilla V. Saulsbury, during a holiday giveaway at work. I'd never been a big soup person but figured these "light, healthy, delicious and beautiful" soups may be worth trying as a sandwich substitute on occasion. I made a few of the recipes - Wild Rice and Corn Chowder with Cajun Spices, Leek and Potato, Split Pea with Caramelized Onions, Roasted Vegetable Minestrone, Bouillabaisse -- and they were everything they were cracked up to be.

I'd never really liked cooking but found I enjoyed making these soups. It was relaxing after a hard day of writing stories about things like Oprah's weight gain and Angelina's anorexia for the supermarket tabloids. And there was an art to creating soup as I tweaked the recipes and came up with some of my own. I'd make big pots, rarely measuring anything, just adding a bit of this and a touch of that as tantalizing aromas filled the kitchen. When I was done and the soup cooled, I'd ladle it into plastic pint containers and freeze them. Each morning, after my bike ride, I'd pick one out to defrost for lunch, and typically supplement it with a small bowl of fresh fruit.

A dozen years later, I'm still doing it. There is something wholesome and comforting in soup, both in the cooking and slurping of it. I don't miss my sandwiches at all, in part because I still have a couple on weekends, albeit with a lot less toxic meat and more veggies, such as avocado, onion, tomato, a variety of greens, sweet and/or hot peppers, and even some homegrown sprouts.

By trading sandwiches for soup five days a week, I'm replacing about the worst meat you can eat and carbs from the bread for what is mostly cooked veggies, often with legumes. I'm eating fewer calories with more nutrients including, quite literally, a shitload of fiber. Fiber is all the stuff your body doesn't digest but keeps your waste removal department running smoothly. And although we can't digest fiber, the little buggies that live within us love it. As you'll soon find out, keeping them well fed can keep you happy and healthy.

The bottom line in switching sandwiches for soups is that I get fewer calories and carbs, which means I can afford more calories and carbs on beer. To drink beer and not gain weight, you have to understand this equation:

Calories taken in minus calories burned equals zero.

Fortunately, the typical human burns between 1,000 and 1,400 calories a day doing nothing more strenuous than breathing. This is technically called the basic metabolic rate. Add another 500 or so if you're not in a coma and sit upright and walk around the house a bit. Exercising will burn more calories, but we'll talk more about that later.

Weight Watchers has the right idea with their calorie-counting plans, but who wants to turn the pleasures of eating (and drinking) into an accounting job? I don't count calories, but I am aware of them. For example, when the boss would bring a box of donuts into the office in the morning, I'd pass figuring I'd rather have a beer after work. Actually, choosing beer over a donut probably saved me fifty calories or more, making the choice a no-brainer.

It's all a matter of being conscious about what you ingest and making smart choices as often as you can. In current pop culture terms, this is called "mindful eating." My choice to shift from sandwiches to soup was easy for me to make and maintain. Now, I'm not saying you should do the same thing, but if not, what kind of shift can you make to give your body better fuel? Just in case it is soup, I'm sharing a few of my favorite recipes with you at the back of this book.

Omelets, Salads And Other Good Stuff

What I do is try to be really good about what I stuff in my mouth on weekdays, so I can cheat some on weekends. Besides my daily soup and fruit, I have an Isagenix whey shake for breakfast (studies show that eating a high-protein breakfast boosts metabolism and keeps you satiated longer into the day than something like a bowl of Frosted Flakes) and sensible dinner. Usually, that includes an omelet once a week.

I have a friend named Darrell, a rugby player in his twenties who'd put on a lot of weight, then lost it. When I asked how he did it, he replied, "I cut out bread and other carbs. I asked myself, 'Can I put it into an omelet?' And if I could, I did, and ate it."

Omelets are great choices because they cram a lot of nutrients into a relatively low-calorie package. There's pretty much an endless variety of what you can use as fillings, and they're delicious.

A few decades ago, eggs were slandered by overzealous heart disease specialists because they have a lot of cholesterol. People were warned to severely limit their consumption of them, or to just go with egg whites, which have no cholesterol.

Well, now the yoke's on them. Research has revealed that dietary cholesterol, the stuff you get from what you eat, has a minimal effect on blood cholesterol levels. Nowadays, eggs are hailed far and wide as a superfood, containing the antioxidants lutein and zeaxanthin, which are good for the eyes; choline, a vitamin-like nutrient good for the brain and nerves; and vitamins A, B and D. One large egg also has about six grams of protein and just seventy-two calories. Add some grilled onions, mushrooms, green pepper and garlic to your omelet along with tomatoes and/or avocado and/or spinach and you up the nutrient density through the roof. As Darrell would attest, you can put almost anything into an omelet and it will taste great, so why not put healthy stuff in there?

Another tasty, healthy dinner is a chef's salad, heavy on the veggies and very light on the meat and cheese. Since iceberg lettuce is perhaps the least nutritious green, I generally go with spring mix and/or romaine with carrots, radishes, celery, tomatoes, peppers of all colors, avocado, artichoke hearts, chickpeas, one slice of ham and/or turkey, feta cheese, hard-boiled egg and pepperoncini for a little bite. The more ingredients the better. Try to top it with homemade dressing as opposed to something store-bought and creamy with tongue-twisting ingredients like propylene glycol alginate and calcium disodium EDTA. Making your own salad dressings is simple – 6 oz. olive oil, 2 oz. balsamic (or apple cider) vinegar, salt, pepper and Mrs. Dash spices, for one -- and much cheaper than buying them at the supermarket.

Other nights I may have grilled salmon, shrimp stir fry, roast chicken or an occasional steak or pork chops, but always with a green salad and a vegetable or two. I like to roast veggies, cutting them into bite-size pieces, tossing them with a little olive oil and spices, and sticking them in the oven for a half-hour or so. Pretty much anything tastes good that way, even Brussels sprouts. If I use rice or pasta, it's always whole grain, which not only has more fiber and nutrients than the refined white varieties but also has a nice nutty flavor.

Making small adjustments, like swapping refined grains for whole, adds up over the long term. And anytime you can eat whole green food, go for it. All the biological energy on Earth comes from the sun, and plants with chlorophyll are the only organisms on the planet that can produce the fuel from that energy that powers our bodies, or the bodies of the animals we eat, at least somewhere along the food chain. The closer you get to the energy source, the better. Green food not only supplies low-glycemic energy but also vitamins, minerals, antioxidants and fiber.

So, basically, I eat really well during the week. Weekends, all bets are off because sometimes you just have to have chicken wings, nachos and fried anything. Despite putting no limits on myself, I still usually end up eating mostly healthy stuff, in part because you just feel better when you're done. The greasy onion rings may taste great in the mouth, but they tend to lay heavy in the gut for a while. Not so with guacamole or hummus. That said, I'm not a fanatic about it. I'm addicted to Cape Cod potato chips, some of the emptiest calories around and loaded with sodium. But I limit myself to one big handful and try my best to savor them, one at a time. I also enjoy some frozen yogurt or, my favorite, an ice cream sandwich for an evening treat. It's OK to eat some nutrition-challenged food so long as you are mindful about it. Be mindful about it and you'll naturally drift to the healthier stuff.

Keeping Your Body's Houseguests Happy

One thing that's important to remember is that you're not just feeding yourself but also about 100 trillion bacteria, viruses, fungi and other microscopic organisms that live with you. You are their ecosystem, their home planet, so to speak. Collectively, these tiny beings you host are called the microbiome. In fact, there's many more of them than there are cells of you in you. And, as I noted while talking about fiber earlier, keeping them happy will help to keep you healthy.

The microbiome flew pretty far under the radar until recent years, and now it's suddenly one of the hottest health topics around. Researchers believe that the balance between beneficial microbes and pathogenic ones is a key to maintaining good health, and imbalances have been linked to everything from Alzheimer's to autism to diabetes to depression and so on.

While I was writing a magazine article about the microbiome, UCLA public health professor William McCarthy illustrated the importance of it right from birth. He said that a human baby lacks the enzymes to digest a class of carbs called oligosaccharides, which are the third most plentiful ingredients (behind fats and lactose) in a mother's breast milk.

"Why would evolution supply fuel for something other than the baby?" Professor McCarthy rhetorically asked during the interview. "It's to feed the baby's microbes. That's how important they are."

Of course, along with the microbiome's newfound importance to health has come various ways to make money off it. Mostly in pill form. If Americans want anything, they want it easy, and what can be easier than swallowing a pill? In this case, the pills are packed with various strains of beneficial bacterial, also known as probiotics. The pills have become a multimillion-dollar industry even though scientists at the government's National Institutes of Health say: "Strong scientific evidence to support specific uses of probiotics for most health conditions is lacking."

More effective than supplements are fermented foods, which have plenty of the friendly little buggers. They include yogurt, sauerkraut, kefir, miso, kombucha and kimchi, most of which taste pretty gnarly. But you know what else is fermented?

Beer.

Unfortunately, our arch-enemy alcohol and the bitter hop acids tend to eradicate most of the bacteria involved with the brewing process. Sorry to pull the rug out from under your hopes that beer can help populate your microbiome with "good" bacteria, but this is not entirely a bad thing since those same bacteria can turn beer bad. Oddly enough, sour beers, which are mildly infected with "good" bacteria, have been gaining in popularity, much to my personal incredulity. But the folks who like it may actually reap some good gut flora from their beer.

There is more to the beer/microbiome connection because our favorite beverage also contains indigestible oligosaccharides, which if you'll recall from a few paragraphs ago help to feed beneficial microbes in babies. They serve the same function in babies who have survived to drinking age, and along with residual yeast and enzymes found in unfiltered beer, like homebrew, help to nourish our bodies' houseguests.

What To Drink When You're Not Drinking Beer

So we can proudly say we not only drink beer for ourselves but also for trillions of others who depend on us. We can say that, even if it's a bit of a stretch. Conversely, the "bad" bacteria in our gut tend to thrive on other liquid refreshment, such as sugar-laden sodas and fruit juices. These are also the most common non-alcoholic sources of liquid calories, and they can add up fast. Since soft drinks have no fiber, they don't do much to fill you up. But the calories they contain are sure to fill you out. I have pretty much cut soda, fruit juices, Gatorade and other hi-cal drinks from my diet because...you guessed it...I'd rather spend those calories on beer.

For many years, I mostly drank either beer or water. But I've expanded my repertoire to include green tea, with just a touch of honey, as well as coffee, with just a splash of cream. They not only offer a little variety, and flavor, to my life, but also a bunch of healthy nutrients.

Green tea is delightfully refreshing, and I've always been partial to green things seeing how my name is Greenberg, and I'm a big fan of St. Patty's Day, if not green beer. Green tea is also on everyone's best foods in the world list, largely due to its uniquely high concentration of an antioxidant called EGCG, aka, epigallocatechin gallate. That, along with other bioactive compounds in green tea, lowers risk of cardiovascular disease, cancer, diabetes, obesity… need I go on? It hits all of the big ones, and even improves brain function so you can better remember important things like where you left your beer. (Can you tell that I often misplace my beer?) Green ice tea is quick to quench a thirst on a hot Florida day. Today happens to be the middle of winter, and it's chilly by South Florida standards, barely cracking seventy degrees. A blustery wind is gusting up to thirty mph, driving the wind chill factor down to a teeth-chattering sixty-five. It's a miracle my fingers aren't too numb from the cold t-o t-y-p-e…

But I can warm up with a nice cup of coffee. Coffee is my other non-water, non-beer go-to. I was never a huge fan and preferred tea, but made the leap over a course of the past year or so. For a while we ground our own beans and brewed it in French presses, which are great unless a) you want quantity or b) you drop them on the counter and break them, which happened recently, one after the other within a week. Now, we have old reliable Mr. Coffee, and he works fine, brewing up to twelve cups at a time according to his pot's imprinted scale, but is really only five or six in real life. During my last month-long beer fast, I subbed iced coffee for beer at my normal beer drinking times, like while watching football, feeding Stella the box turtle in her habitat, and hanging out in the hammocks on a lazy afternoon. Like beer, coffee has very strong and complex flavors that make it interesting to the palate. It's very satisfying and, as it turns out, incredibly healthy. Researchers in several studies have found that people who drink coffee are less likely to die than those who don't, and pretty much the more the better. Dr. Sammy Saab, a professor of hepatology at UCLA's David Geffen School of Medicine, told me that coffee protects the liver, which can be damaged – sometimes critically -- by alcohol. On the downside, you don't catch a buzz from it.

Moving on, I recently tried some flavored sparkling water brands that are as fizzy and sweet as soda, but weigh in at zero calories. There's something unnatural about that, not to mention the red dye #40. And they have the same synthetic aftertaste as artificial sweeteners. So I think I'll pass. But it may work for you, and if you save 140 calories compared to a can of Coke, that's 140 you have in the bank for beer. I've come to prefer sparkling water with minimal "natural" flavoring, which lacks the sweetness and food dyes but retains a satisfying fizz.

The more smart choices you make about what you consume besides beer, the more beer your body will tolerate.

Bad choices include sodas, fruit juices, sports drinks and all other heavily sweetened fluids, including those with artificial sweeteners; cold cuts; cakes, pies, donuts, sweet rolls and anything from Entenmann's; bacon (sorry); potato chips; fried food;

pizza; factory-farmed meat and poultry products; cookies; candy; white bread, white rice and white pasta; and anything that is highly processed.

Good choices include whole fruit and vegetables (organic if possible, and especially greens, avocados, broccoli, onions, garlic, hot peppers, carrots and beets); mushrooms; wild-caught fish; fermented food; oatmeal (not instant); beans and other legumes; eggs (with yolks); spices (excluding salt because we get so much of it without trying); and even air-popped popcorn (hold the so-called "butter").

Then we have some in-between choices, which are foods that are okay in moderation when coming from a healthy environment, which doesn't include places that keep animals in crowded, unnatural conditions and/or spikes feed with antibiotics and/or hormones. These foods include meat (grass-fed when possible); free-range poultry; whole grains (which have lots of nutrients and fiber but are still high in carbs); and dairy from grass-fed animals.

I still eat food from each of these three food groups, but have shifted much of the load to the healthiest stuff. One trick is to stop buying the junk. If you buy apples and oranges instead of cookies and cakes, that's all you have to turn to when needing to feed your sweet-tooth. So you'll eat the fruit, and it will be sweet and satisfying, and loaded with vitamins, minerals antioxidants, fiber, yaddah, yaddah yaddah… Keep your cupboard and fridge stocked with the good stuff, and then it won't hurt so much on those infrequent occasions when you down a few brews at the county fair and wind up stuffing your face with corndogs and funnel cake.

To summarize, the fewer calories you spend on solid food, the more you have available for beer. So try to eat a lot of foods that are densely packed with nutrition and less junk food that works out to be empty calories. By all means cheat on occasion, but be aware that you are cheating and try to limit the damage. And please don't be like my wife Nora, who can stick steadfastly to a diet, exercise regimen and anything else for a good amount of time until she slips up once, at which point she histrionically throws her hands up in the air, announces that she's blown it and proceeds to go hog-wild for a while as if to make up for lost time. If you slip up, fuhgeddaboutit and get back on track.

I don't do all this specifically so I can get away with drinking more beer, but that is one of the end results.

Chapter 7
Earning Your Beer

The alarm goes off at 6:34 a.m…"you gotta move…you gotta move"…that old Rolling Stones song echoes through your head as you struggle to rouse your still deactivated body…"you gotta move…you gotta move"…

Some days are easier than others. Some days you're already awake or just about to be; other days you're dead to the world. On this day, you feel on par with a zombie, minus the appetite for human brains. You know that if you can manage to slip one leg out from under the covers to land a foot on the floor, you can ease yourself out of bed and stagger naked down the hallway to the living room, where late last night you left your weathered Columbia Eagle River Swim Shorts, whatever t-shirt you'd worn the day before, and clean socks on the easy chair. You pull on the shorts and shirt, then sit in the chair to don your socks and old sneakers, which you use instead of new ones because you never know when you're going to be drenched by a sudden rain shower while pedaling a bicycle around Boca Raton.

Once dressed, you grab your cell phone and earbuds, shuffle into to kitchen to fill your spill-proof mug with ice water and head out to the shed in the backyard, where you park your bike. You used to keep it in the detached laundry room closer to the house, but in the middle of the morning on the Fourth of July a few years back, someone stole it from there. There were five people and two dogs in the house at the time. In other words, the thief got lucky, and you didn't. So now you park your bike in the shed you unfailingly keep locked even though a ton of people know the key is hidden under the sundial (not really, but somewhere nearby). You roll out your "classic" Schwinn road bike, a gold Le Tour

Luxe from the 1980s. The frame is rusty and the wrapping on the curved handlebars looks like something a 5,000-year-old mummy would wear. You got it off Craig's List after your last bike was stolen, figuring that a beat-up old bike is less likely to be stolen, despite that fact that all of your bikes have been kind of beat up and most have been stolen. Though it looks like crap, you keep your Schwinn relatively well tuned with occasional squirts of WD-40 in vital moving parts and air in the tires.

Some days it's dark when you hit the road, but this time of year there's the budding light of sunrise. Some days, you ride through the mostly deserted streets of downtown Boca Raton, over the drawbridge and north or south alongside the beach on the redundantly-named stretch of road known as A1A. Some days, you ride through Royal Palm, the oldest gated community in South Florida, replete with stucco-walled, barrel tile-roofed mansions lining the Intracoastal waterway or a pristine golf course. Today you cruise along El Rio Trail, a thin slice of wilderness on the eastern flank of Florida Atlantic University. It runs alongside thirty-foot-wide El Rio Canal, hence the name. As you pedal along, you see some regulars on the trail, like the stocky guy who power-walks clad in the same bilious green guayabera every day, a Chinese woman who didn't acknowledge you for about five years but recently began casting you a reserved smile, and a woman kicking back on a beach cruiser with phone in hand, single earplug in ear and yakking away to someone or, these days, something.

But most of the way, you're alone on the shady asphalt pathway. Even the critters are scarce, including South Florida's seemingly limitless species of bugs. The iguanas that have invaded these parts from points south aren't up yet, because they like the heat of the day rather than the chill of dawn. A few little birds flutter about, wrens, warblers, sparrows or something. A heron stands on spindly legs by the canal and white ibises scurry about at the edge of a meadow, poking their long orange beaks into the turf. When something dead is around, you see turkey vultures turning graceful arcs in the sky.

You once saw a gray fox. It was sitting in the middle of El Rio Trail when you rounded a bend, looking your way as though expecting you. At first you thought it was a small dog, or big cat. But then it flashed its distinctive fluffy fox tail as it bounded away and into a thicket of Brazilian peppers. That happened once in twenty years, which makes it memorable.

Although you can't see most of the animal life around you, it still gives you energy. And there's more energy in the trees and scrub brush flanking the trail. The sun finally peeks over the horizon, casting everything in a fleeting golden glow. You listen to Pandora, which streams tunes from your favorite musicians through your cellphone, never quite getting over the awe of being able to carry a juke box in your pocket. Sometimes you think about things, the day ahead or behind. But mostly you think about nothing other than pedaling along and taking it all in. Life is beautiful, peaceful and uncomplicated, at least for the first thirty or forty minutes of your day.

Getting An Early Start

I hope you enjoyed coming along on one of my morning bike rides. In truth, it is more pleasant to write about than actually do, as exercise is inherently uncomfortable, and often what I think about along the way is how much farther I have to go before I'm done. But once I round the final bend, whistle to let the dog know I'm home, and dismount on the gated patio to a spirited if somewhat slobbery greeting, I feel terrific.

There's not one vestige of sleep left in my body, which is totally energized despite having just spent a lot of energy. I have no idea how many calories I've burned, though figure it's surely enough to make up for one or two beers later on. Besides the calories expended, there are other physiological factors triggered by exercise that ramp up the metabolism for hours afterward, even when sitting inertly in front of a computer. This higher metabolism rate burns more calories which, of course, frees up those calories for other things, such as beer.

Exercise is really one of the top things you can do for your body. In fact, if scientists could come up with a pill that replaces exercise, it would be the best supplement ever. It would increase blood flow, burn fat, build lean muscle mass, strengthen bones, release hormones to improve mood and lower stress, detoxify the body, aid sleep, invigorate sex, promote healthy aging, and boost longevity. But such a pill has not yet been invented, and likely won't be anytime soon. So our only option is to set aside at least a half-hour or so each day to ride a bike, or jog, or swim, or even just walk briskly. You can play games, like tennis or basketball, or take classes, like Zumba or spinning, or do a bit of everything to break up the monotony. The important thing is to do something.

I know what a lot of you are thinking: "Between work, the kids' activities and everything else I've got to do in life, I just don't have the time to exercise." To which I say: "Find it." I don't naturally wake up at 6:34 a.m. I started doing it because at one point in my life (circa 1997) I also was having trouble squeezing exercise into my daily schedule, which included a fifty-mile daily commute between Boca Raton and

Key Biscayne in some of the most heavily congested traffic east of Los Angeles. Before adjusting my schedule, I'd normally arise at 7:30 a.m. so I could have my tea, read the paper and still get to work in time to do my 10 a.m. to 6 p.m. shift as a general assignment reporter for *The Islander News*. By the time I got home at 7 p.m. or later, and had dinner, washed the dishes, spent some quality time with my wife and then young son, and walked the dog, well, it was time to go to bed. There simply weren't enough hours in the day for exercise, so I made more hours by waking up earlier, even though I'd never really been a "morning person."

It can be a bit tough to get going, especially when it's still dark at 6:34 a.m. (initially I was going to set the alarm for 6:30 but overshot it, figured 6:34 was close enough and never bothered to change it). But once I'm on the road, my body doesn't care about the time of day too much. And it's better to ride a bike on the streets of Boca Raton before the traffic picks up because there are a lot of crappy drivers here, and as we all know, whether the cyclist hits the car or the car hits the cyclist, it's going to be bad for the cyclist.

Another good thing about exercising first thing is that, notwithstanding a spot of rain, nothing will get in the way. Later in the day, there could be unforeseen problems with work, family, traffic or digestive tract from those truck tacos you scarfed at lunch, any of which could usurp your exercise time. Do it first thing in the morning and you're less likely to miss it.

While any type of exercise is better than none, one type is particularly good for not only stimulating the metabolism but also fitting into almost any schedule. It's called high intensity interval training (HIIT) and consists of short bursts of all-out effort interspersed with a slower recovery pace. For those of you who remember anything from high school biology, it's the difference between aerobic and anaerobic exercise. For those of you who don't, it doesn't really matter. The point is that if you can include some high-intensity exercise that really gets your heart rate going, you will get much more benefit out of the time you spend working out.

An effective HIIT workout can be done in as little as fifteen minutes and will reap the same, or more, benefits than an hour of moderate-paced aerobic exercise. The simplest involves doing three thirty-second sets of five calisthenics – such as push-ups, lunges, jumping jacks, squats and crunches – as fast as you can with thirty-second rests between each set. Or, like me, you can incorporate HIIT into your regular regimen of running, swimming, biking, skating or other aerobic activity. In my case, on my bike ride a couple of days a week, I do thirty seconds of all-out pedaling, then throttle back for a couple of minutes, then go all-out for another thirty seconds, and so on throughout my seven- or eight-mile loop.

HIIT training is even more uncomfortable than regular exercise. But it's also one of the few ways we know to trigger a process called mitochondria biogenesis. Excuse me while I get slightly technical here, but mitochondria health is directly related to processing calories, including the ones you get from drinking beer. These organelles serve as tiny generators that power our bodies' cells, and HIIT training is one of the only ways known to create new ones. As we age, our mitochondria tend to dysfunction, which is one reason why old people often complain about having no energy. That lack of energy also makes it harder for cells to maintain themselves and they break down, eventually leading to saggy skin, achy joints, hearing loss and other hallmarks of aging, including a variety of chronic and often deadly conditions, such as cancer, Alzheimer's and heart disease.

Obviously, all of these consequences of mitochondria dysfunction can put a crimp in your beer drinking pleasures. But you can battle Father Time with sweat. In a landmark study published in the journal *Cell Metabolism* in 2017, researchers at the esteemed Mayo Clinic in Minnesota found that HIIT training appeared to "slow down aging at a cellular level by reversing deterioration of mitochondria." More healthy mitochondria mean more energy, which means better overall health, which means more capacity to enjoy more beer for more years of your life.

Experts also recommend doing some resistance training, such as weight lifting, to help maintain muscle mass, which dissipates with age. Since weights always seem to tweak my back, I do old fashioned calisthenics: mostly push-ups, planks, deep knee bends and squat thrusts, also known as burpees, which is one of the more silly-sounding words in the English language along with filibuster, nincompoop, lollygag, cockamamie, gobbledygook, codpiece and near-beer. I perform these exercises during breaks in my writing endeavors, as I often need a respite from thinking so hard to make my writing seem spontaneous and effortless. Sometimes, I surf around the Internet to check out Facebook, CNN or Pornhub, and sometimes I get off my butt and do some calisthenics. While blasts of exercise may not be as much fun as scrutinizing the astonishing assortment of human mating habits on Pornhub, they do increase the flow of oxygen and blood throughout the *whole* body to both nourish cells and eliminate their waste. Numerous studies link sitting uninterrupted for long periods of time with obesity, high blood pressure, high cholesterol and an increased risk of death from heart disease or cancer, not to mention a sore butt. Our brainy friends at the Mayo Clinic advise taking a break from sitting every thirty minutes. And you're better off cranking out a few pushups than fetching a snack from the fridge.

Another good idea is to get a dog. Scientists say that any kind of pet helps to improve longevity, but I like dogs, in part because they take me for a lot of walks. Typically, we go strolling around the neighborhood after dinner, which helps to burn off some of the calories I've just consumed. Thigh muscles, in particular, really gobble up the glucose when engaged, leaving less to turn into fat. An evening walk is also a good stress-buster, unless your wife comes along and keeps talking about all the things you need to do or shouldn't have done.

Beer Break

I have before me a glass of Sierra Nevada Pale Ale, a beer that continues to astound me because it is so commonplace and moderately-priced, yet so sublime. Created by onetime homebrewer Ken Grossman in the early 1980s, the classic ale not only endures but thrives. As my thirty-something nephew Matt says: "Sierra Nevada Pale Ale is my if-I-was-stranded-on-a-desert-island-and-could-only-have-one-beer beer." It is pale ale perfection, though often overlooked as we constantly seek out the exotic. Made with American Cascade hops and top quality two-row malts, it's simple yet satisfying, refreshing yet rich. It has the balls of an IPA but more of a nip than bite of bitterness. And at 5.6 percent ABV, you can drink a fair share of it on a hot day, but it's also good for sipping around the campfire at night.

Sierra Nevada was a pioneer of the craft beer industry, taking on Anheuser-Busch, Coors, Miller and the other heavyweights, and carving out a niche market that's now worth close to $1 billion. It's American entrepreneurship at its best, as are the thousands of smaller breweries that have followed its path. Unlike the unimaginative big boys, who churned out the same limited line-ups of taste-challenged lager for decades, Sierra Nevada continues to innovate with countless special releases to complement a varied slate of year-round and seasonal brews. They offer a Beer Camp to teach others the craft, and some years produce a mixed 12-pack with the best Beer Camp recipes. They collaborate with other breweries for some of their special releases and, being from California, are socially conscious. For example, in the wake of the catastrophic Camp Fire of 2018 that destroyed much of Butte County, Sierra Nevada organized a fundraiser. Enlisting the help of some 1,400 other breweries, they produced Resilience Butte County Proud IPA, and reportedly donated 100 percent of the sales of some 17,000 barrels to a relief fund.

So, this beer's for you, Ken Grossman, and Fritz Maytag from Anchor Brewing, Jim Koch from Samuel Adams and the rest of the early craft brewers who have changed the beer drinking landscape of America, for the better.

Stretching The Limit

One aspect of my daily physical regimen I've yet to

mention is stretching, which has little to do with bolstering the body to maximize tolerable beer consumption but is still important. Stretching is widely overlooked by many diehard exercisers. However, it's hard to enjoy anything if various parts of your body wind up twisted or contorted to the point that you have trouble walking over to the fridge to fetch a beer or hoisting a pint with gnarled hands. Stretching can help prevent, or at least minimize the effects of arthritis, tendonitis and other conditions that limit range of motion. To make an analogy, if you never open your basement door for twenty years, it becomes tougher, if not impossible, to open because debris settles in the hinges and all around the door. But if you open it as far as it will go just once every day, it will continue to open easily, even two decades down the road. Same goes with your body. Keep stretching it out, and it will resist tightening up.

Because I was one of an ever-increasing number of journalists who got laid off from regular jobs in recent years, I now make my own schedule as a freelance writer and thus have the luxury to spend about forty-five minutes stretching out every day after my morning bike ride. As a former high school gymnast, I use many of the same stretches now as I did then. They resemble yoga poses and focus on legs and pelvis but also cover back, shoulders, neck, fingers and even eyes, which I roll around in their sockets ten times each way every day. I do that because I once read that exercising the eye muscles will help combat age-related vision impairment, which it hasn't, seeing how I need stronger glasses every few years anyway. But I suppose it can't hurt, and eye-rolling is easier than pushups.

After stretching most every part of my body, I use a foam roller to help massage and hydrate fascia, the gauze-like connective tissue that envelopes muscles and organs. The fascia stabilizes our internal structure, but it can get compromised by various tensions, ranging from sitting in a chair all day to toxins in the food we eat to stress from getting stuck in traffic to playing a game of rugby. And when that happens, it can inhibit movement and organ function and cause pain.

"When you wake up in the morning and feel stiff, the dehydrated fascia is what's causing that stiffness," says therapist Sue Hitzmann, co-author of a wonderful book about fascia care called *The MELT Method*. "When you rehydrate the fascia, you feel great and have a happy body."

After MELTing a bit with a foam roller, I take a few minutes to do deep breathing exercises. Like the rest of the body, it's good to stretch out the lungs by inhaling as much air as possible, holding it for a few counts, then slowly letting it out until your lungs are as deflated as you can get them. I wait until my body feels as if it is collapsing into itself before talking another deep breath, and do that five times.

I wind up my morning workout by hanging upside-down on an inversion table for ten minutes. Turning ass-over-tea kettle shakes up both the circulatory and lymphatic systems and decompresses the spine. While it feels great to me, it is not for everyone, especially people with glaucoma, a condition of elevated pressure in the eyeball which, as you might imagine, doesn't go well with hanging upside down. Ironically, hanging upside down can also hurt the spine, which is the very thing it is meant to help. We once had a couple of Jamaican rugby players stay with us for a while. They were super-fit and worked out a lot. But when one of them tried the inversion table, it hurt his back to the point he had to miss a game or two. So definitely ask your healthcare provider before using an inversion device. And try one out before buying because they obviously aren't for everyone.

By the time I turn right-side up again and head into the kitchen for my morning protein shake and cup of tea, my body feels both relaxed and enervated, and I have a happy buzz going thanks to the feel-good endorphin hormones released through exercise. It's barely eight o'clock in the morning, and I've already accomplished what may be the most important task of the day as far as my physical well-being goes. It will be several hours before I have my first beer, but I've already earned it.

A Word About Hydration

After working up a good sweat, it's important to replenish lost fluids. For most of humankind's existence, hydration consisted of plain water, which still works fine today. In 1965, researchers at the University of Florida developed a drink to help their football players rehydrate during games. The team was called the Gators, and the drink was initially dubbed "Gator-Aid," which marketing people changed to "Gatorade." Along with water, Gatorade contains added electrolytes - sodium, chloride, potassium, magnesium and calcium - to replenish what football players and other athletes sweat out.

Gatorade also contains nearly as much added sugar as soda, which was probably beneficial to the Gators. During games, they used up a lot of glucose for energy, and the body can only store a finite amount of it, so they needed more to burn. But most of us, and football players after the game, don't need all of that added sugar any more than we need the petroleum-based food dyes that give sports drinks their unnaturally vibrant colors, such as Gatorade's classic "anti-freeze" green. Gatorade has spawned a whole industry of mostly vibrant-colored sports drinks, which do more to support our nation's ongoing obesity epidemic than support the replenishment of lost electrolytes.

So, you're better off to rehydrate with filtered water after your workout. But there is another option gaining popularity, and you won't believe what it is.

Beer.

Well, kinda. It's not the regular stuff but rather a non-alcoholic variety that has caught on bigtime in Germany, the country with the largest per capita consumption of beer (actually bier) in the world. Since the alcohol in beer is a diuretic and causes water elimination, the reason why you pee a lot when imbibing, it's removed. What's left is lower in sugar than the standard sports drinks but also contains phenols, plant-based compounds that help to reduce inflammation and fight infection. As we've noted before, beer is also a rarely rich source of silicon, which helps to build strong bones, as well as those indigestible prebiotic oligosaccharides that are good for your gut bacteria. German sports beer drinks also have added electrolytes similar to Gatorade to replace those that get sweated out.

Of course, the drawback to non-alcoholic beer is that you can't catch a buzz from it, thus leaving the world a little less warm and fuzzy, especially to the loser of the sports competition. But innovative American brewer Sam Calagione, co-founder of Delaware-based Dogfish Head Brewery, has created a supposedly hydrating alcoholic brew called SeaQuench Ale. Ingredients are said to include special strains of potassium-rich barley, sea salts from Maine and Chesapeake Bay, and black limes from Egypt, Turkey and Guatemala. It reportedly boasts a tart, slightly sour flavor, a modest 140 calories per 12-ounce bottle and a respectable 4.9 percent ABV.

Even though it's kind of like having your cake and drinking it, too, I'm not sure I'd like SeaQuench Ale, seeing how I don't like my beer on the sour side and have an unusually (for me) hostile attitude towards mixing beer and lime. During the years I lived in the San Diego area (1978-82), Corona beer was like the Old Milwaukee of Mexico. It was the cheapest beer around (as I recall, six-packs went for $1.50) and tasted it, and we used to joke about the Mexicans not being able to afford tinted bottles. I left California to travel abroad for a couple of years, and when I came back to the States, I was stunned to discover that someone had decided to stick a wedge of lime in the mouth of a Corona bottle and start marketing it as a premium beer, with a price to match. That ruined me for beer with lime, not to mention I just don't like how it tastes.

Besides, I'm not really sure you have to go to all of that trouble. Despite what the science may say about beer and hydration, it seems to work fine for me. There have been numerous times when, after playing eighty minutes of rugby, I slaked my thirst with nothing but beer for hours and it always made me feel better, not worse, at least until the morning. Furthermore, when I drink a lot of beer, I have to piss a lot. When you're dehydrated, the experts say your pee is relatively dark. When I drink beer, my pee is light, eventually running pretty near clear. So I not only appear to be well hydrated but am also flushing my…

Hmmmm. It seems our discussion about exercise has devolved into one about piss. Allow me to apologize, and let's move on.

Chapter 8
The Beer-Lover's Lifestyle

There's little doubt that diet and exercise are the two main pillars supporting good health and thus vital to being able to enjoy the consumption of our favorite beverage. However, there are a lot of other factors that contribute mightily to health and longevity, including some that can even sabotage a lot of the good you do for yourself by eating right and working out.

Lifestyle covers a lot of territory. It's basically everything you do, and even think as far as attitude goes. Most of us get pretty set in our ways, and those routines tend to become even more rigid as we age and find ourselves less willing to change. We get comfy in our own little world, living in the same home, hanging out with the same group of people, going to the same places to socialize, and even settling on a favorite beer or ten. You may feel happy and satisfied, but ultimately it's like swimming endless laps around Stagnation Pond. Most of us crave more but are too lazy or scared to pursue it. We don't like getting outside our comfort zone because it can be, well, uncomfortable. But just like exercise, you need to get a bit uncomfortable to grow stronger, and wiser.

While studying journalism (along with rugby, coeds and beer) in college, I once covered a speech given by Dustin Hoffman, a great actor who downs Olympia beer in his breakthrough movie *The Graduate* as he commences his decline from promising college grad to MILF debauchery. I remember it being a great speech, but the only part that has stuck with me for more than forty years is how he described change.

"I hated asparagus when I was young," he said. "Now, I love it. The fact that you can hate asparagus one day, and love it another day…well, isn't that terrific?"

Although I personally had yet to turn the corner on asparagus, I got the point. Even a stupid little change like that was enough to get Hoffman's eyes gleaming, and his enthrallment was contagious. Life is all about change, forging ever forward into new territory, and adapting your mind and body to meet the challenges. We continually face new challenges, especially as we age. We have to adapt to stay healthy and strong enough to enjoy a bit too much fine ale on occasion. Try to tweak your lifestyle here and there. Fine tune it to be in harmony with your body, and see how far it can take you along the path of well-being.

Blue Zones

National Geographic writer Dan Buettner has studied this lifestyle stuff in relation to communities with the highest concentration of centenarians, who can potentially drink beer for eight decades or more. Initially, he identified five of them scattered around the world and dubbed them "Blue Zones." The people living in Blue Zones shared several characteristics, including:

- Natural movement: They don't need to ride a bike every morning because they get plenty of exercise just living their normal, mostly agrarian lives, gardening, house cleaning and transporting themselves around without much, if any, mechanical help.

- Eating Beans: Beans, beans are good for the heart…and, apparently the rest of the body. Rather than meat anchoring most meals, Blue Zone people eat beans, which have protein, loads of fiber and lots of other healthy compounds without any real downside other than the more you eat them, the more you fart. Generally, they also eat homegrown veggies and just one serving of meat a week. And they don't stuff themselves, especially at evening meals.
- Sense of Purpose: They all have a reason to get up in the morning, whether tending to their garden, or great-grandchildren, or creative endeavor. If you have something to live for, you live longer.
- Social connections: They live in places where you know your neighbors, and often hang out with them. Neighbors in these places are likely to have healthy habits, which studies show to be as contagious as unhealthy habits. They are also very family-oriented, often living in multi-generational homes.
- Relaxing: They know that the body and mind both need some time to just kick back and not do much of anything. They achieve this in different ways – prayer, meditation, napping - but all of them know it's important to unwind and give the body a break from those damaging stress hormones.

- Beer: Well, maybe not specifically. But with just one exception, all of the Blue Zones people drink moderately, the same one-to-two drinks a day that the AMA recommends.

My favorite Blue Zones story took place in Loma Linda, California, home to a community of Seventh-day Adventists. Members of this Christian sect are vegetarian teetotalers (both of which are likely to increase longevity), and like Jews, observe the Sabbath on Saturday rather than Sunday (no data on whether that increases longevity, but observing Sabbath on any day may help out if it doesn't). One doctor in his nineties needed a new wooden fence on his property and, finding estimates too high, did the job himself, including the backbreaking work of digging holes for the posts. The next day he landed in the hospital for open-heart surgery. But he wasn't the one on the table. He was the one performing the operation. Even after hanging up his scalpel at age ninety-six, Dr. Ellsworth Wareham continued to drive and garden right up until his death at 104.

Although that's a great story, Dr. Wareham is somewhat irrelevant to our discussion seeing how he didn't partake in even one or two beers a day. But if he did, he no doubt would have enjoyed them, right along with his driving and gardening, until he died.

Fortunately, you don't need to be a Seventh-day Adventist to live a long healthy life. Case in point is Stamatis Moraitis, a Greek immigrant laborer who was diagnosed with terminal lung cancer at age sixty and given just nine months to live. Having settled in Boynton Beach, Florida, he decided to return to his birth home on the Greek island of Ikaria to die, in part because the funeral would be cheaper, leaving more money for his soon-to-be widow. Then a funny thing happened. He didn't die. With no therapy other than good food, fresh air, no particular schedule, lots of friends and long nights sipping local wine and playing dominoes in the town tavern, Moraitis was still going strong at age ninety-seven, more than three decades after resettling on Ikaria, which is another of Buettner's Blue Zones.

Busting Stress

One of the secrets to longevity, which the Blue Zoners seem to have mastered, is eliminating a lot of stress. They aren't driven to have more than the Joneses, or Warehams, or Moraitises. They aren't pressed for time or constantly checking to see how many "likes" their last Facebook post garnered. They enjoy simple pleasures, and I urge you to seek some time in your busy day to do the same.

One place I find it is by the turtle pen, a fenced-in niche at the northeastern corner of my Boca Raton property. I go there to feed Stella, a Florida box turtle, which is technically illegal to keep as a pet in this part of the country. I found her when I saw Banyan, a former family dog, chewing on something I thought was a rock but turned out to be a young turtle. The front of her shell was pretty much chewed off and, surprisingly to me, bleeding. Nora, Glen and I nursed Stella back to health and she's become part of the family, which also includes our current canine Roxanne, birds Baba (a sun conure with an attitude) and Olaf (a parakeet with the birdie equivalent of a hare-lip), and a bearded dragon lizard named Klaus.

Stella is the only one who lives outside. Her habitat is a nice wooden pen with plenty of room to roam, go for a swim in her concrete birdbath pond and occasionally interact with humans and superworms, though in much different manners.

After a hard day's toil as a freelance writer, I often grab a beer (homebrew if I have it) and head out to the turtle pen around dusk. The light is the best then, and the tropical skies in Boca Raton are regularly postcard-quality material. I could further describe the parade of puffy clouds drifting lazily across the sky, languid rays from the setting sun transforming them into vibrant canvases ablaze in a cornucopia of colors: tangerine, fuchsia and magenta…but this is not a romance book. Still, it's pretty and serene. I sit on a wooden bench, feed Stella some superworms, drink a beer and totally unwind. Ironically, this part of our property is the most exposed. Through a four-foot chain-link fence, I can see people driving or biking past, or walking their dogs, or just themselves. An occasional skateboarder rolls by because we are situated on the highest point of Boca Raton (54 feet above sea level) and there's a bona fide hill on aptly named High Street, whose sign regularly gets stolen.

For the most part, I see the other people, but they don't see me amidst the plants and trees. Along with the turtle pen, there's a raised garden. Things don't grow too well in it because the neighbor's mango tree blocks the morning sun and an ancient sea grape on our side takes over after that. But some pretty wildflowers spring up, mainly yellow and white and purple ones. For a short while, we had a pair of water turtles named Moe and Joe living there. But they had an unfortunate run-in with raccoons and, sadly, are now just shells of their former selves.

Still, there's a lot of life around. We have a variety of bugs and birds, gray squirrels, iguanas, little anoles, and an occasional snake. I bring some meal worms for the anoles, who dart out of nowhere to snatch them. Bold ones will take them right from my hand. Birds come and go depending on the season. Blue jays, cardinals, doves, mockingbirds…little red-headed woodpeckers sometimes peck on a coconut palm, or a flock of green parrots congregate in a neighbor's pine, squawking away.

I breathe it all in, and try to sip my beer as slowly as possible. I'm so relaxed. My mind wanders, exploring uncharted corners of my creativity. Great ideas pop in and out of my head. Some I will use. Others don't seem so great the next day.

No matter how slowly I drink my beer, it goes too fast. But even one brew is enough to mellow my mood and bolster my confidence. Fears about life's various tribulations fade away. For a few brief shining moments, I have no worries. It's a beautiful feeling I get out by the turtle pen. Everyone should have something like that, because you need a place to drink a beer in peace, and feel whole.

If you don't have a turtle pen or some other kind of sanctuary-type place to chill out, there are many other ways to unwind. Meditation, yoga and exercise are all great stress-busters, as is alcohol. In fact, scientists believe that alcohol's stress-reducing properties are a big reason why moderate consumption of the Demon is associated with longevity. Tragically, most of the beer-lovers I know (including me) are hardly moderate in their consumption, thus negating the longevity benefits of its stress reduction.

Another way to help beat stress is by taking adaptogens, an amazing collection of herbs that help bring the body into hormonal balance. I found out about them through Isagenix, the supplement company that also turned me on to intermittent fasting. Ginseng is probably the best known adaptogen, but others include ashwagandha, rhodiola rosea, astragalus, eleuthero, schisandra, maca and holy basil. They're called "adaptogens" because they adapt to give your body what it needs, generally in terms of hormone regulation. Most have been used in Ayurveda and other traditional medicines for thousands of years, but they are not commonly used in the States, in part because the pharmaceutical companies can't patent them.

During the Cold War, the Soviets researched adaptogens in their endless quest to get an edge over the West, and they published more than a thousand studies about them. Basically, the Soviets found that the herbs helped everyone from soldiers to ballerinas improve their overall performance.

The plants tend to live in harsh climates, and the same compounds that help them survive stressors like high altitude, cold weather and arid climes can also help humans cope with stressors like horrible bosses, whiny kids and traffic jams -- kind of like beer, but without the alcohol.

Sleep

"Ah, sleep," utters W.C. Fields in *My Little Chickadee*. "The most beautiful experience in life – except drink."

Actually, sleep and drink often go together, especially when you've had way too much of the latter and find yourself suddenly asleep, hopefully in a friendly bed as opposed to an all-night diner booth, bus, subway, sidewalk, gutter or serial killer's lair. In truth, alcohol is not a good sleep aid. While it may help you to conk off quickly, your slumber will soon turn restless, disrupting the deep sleep and REM (rapid eye movement) stages your body and brain need for maintenance and repair. Researchers also find that a nightcap or two will make you more likely to snore, which probably won't bother you at the time but could wind up bothering anyone sharing your bed, who will bother you about it come morning.

Sleep is important for beer drinkers because it helps to keep you trim. And the trimmer you are, the more beer you can drink. Primarily, it is a tale of two hormones: ghrelin and leptin. Ghrelin stimulates appetite and fat production while leptin signals that you are full and can start ramping up your energy output. When you don't sleep well, ghrelin levels rise and leptin levels sink. You not only will be hungrier but also crave fatty, high-calorie foods, such as donuts (no coincidence that they are a popular breakfast item). That can lead to an accumulation of visceral fat that is hidden deep in the abdomen. If you remember from our chapter about beer bellies, visceral fat wraps around the liver, kidneys, pancreas and other organs, inhibiting their function while spewing out inflammatory agents that increase risk of diabetes, heart disease, cancer and many other ailments.

So a lack of quality sleep can work below the surface to undermine healthy endeavors. It's best to skip the nightcap, or replace it with something truly sleep inducing, such as chamomile tea or Conan O'Brien.

One problem with deep sleeping is that it gets harder as we age, which is why older people have trouble sleeping through the night. Typically, that has to do with the hormone melatonin, which regulates the circadian rhythm (sleep-wake cycle). Like many other vital compounds, our body's production of melatonin drops with age.

The good news is that melatonin comes in supplement form. I take a spray version of it (supposedly more bioactive than the pills) every night about a half-hour before lights-out and, whether a placebo effect or not, I seem to sleep pretty soundly. In other exciting melatonin news, researchers at the University of Granada in Spain found that melatonin also stimulates the transformation of lardy "white" visceral fat into healthy "beige" fat, at least in lab rats. The difference is that beige fat is packed with mitochondria that burn calories whereas white fat just stores them inertly. So, theoretically, melatonin can help you lose weight while you sleep, especially if you are a lab rat.

There are a lot of good reasons to get at least seven hours of quality sleep a night. Among other things, you'll be less likely to gain weight and accumulate excess quantities of that nasty visceral fat, leaving room for a little more beer in your life.

Social Connections

The concept of "social connections" has changed dramatically over the course of my lifetime, most notably in the last decade or so. Now, we often connect through social media on a device as opposed to face-to-face. It's an evolution. We are inevitably becoming more machinelike while our machines become more humanlike, transformations that will probably progress until we can't tell one from the other, like Arnold Schwarzenegger in *The Terminator*.

I have 511 Facebook friends, many of whom I actually know and like, in the traditional sense of having warm and fuzzy feelings for them, especially after a few beers. Others, I have little or no recognition of.

I'm not a big fan of social media. I've found that I can either experience life fully or try to capture it, but can't really do both at the same time. As I've already mentioned, I spent nearly two years wandering around Europe and the Middle East in the early 1980s and wound up shooting a grand total of seven rolls of film, one that was bad. Despite the relatively meager quantity of photos, I have a representative record of my trip, including snapshots of me with hair tousled by the wind on the summit of the Matterhorn; standing alongside my trusty Honda 250cc motorcycle in Amsterdam; ferrying past a medieval castle along the Rhine; galloping a horse across the desert sands in Giza; and my then Swiss girlfriend Uschi posing topless on the Sinai Peninsula. While I missed capturing a lot of other things in photos, the best (and worst) things stick in my mind without needing anything material to spark the memory.

Nowadays, I can't talk to my wife on road trips because she's Facebooking, delving into the lives of others while missing what's happening in ours. I think the internet has created a serious disconnect between people that is going to manifest itself in some pretty bizarre ways as time goes on. There's no stopping it, but we also need that human connection, to see and touch and feel the warmth that you can't get in the same way online.

And that's a bit weird, coming from me. I've always been a bit of a lone wolf, often traveling on my own, happy not having to worry about anyone else. Nora is the complete opposite, a party person who thinks in terms of groups. Our differences are one reason we make a good couple, though those same differences probably would have kept us from ever hooking up through online dating.

We have nice circle of friends, including neighbors, Nora's "krewe" from New Orleans (where she spent her formative years), pals from work and others, but largely rugby-related. The camaraderie amongst rugby players is legendary. It transcends borders, races, gender, politics and age. When I traveled around, local ruggers in Britain, Wales, Denmark and Germany welcomed me to their world, sharing their lives, homes and beers with me. When I landed in Fort Lauderdale, I knew no one except my parents. But after joining the Knights RFC (Rugby Football Club), I suddenly had dozens of friends, many of whom I'm still close to decades later. And I continue to make new friends through the club, some of them young enough to be my grandchildren.

When I hit sixty-six late last year, I decided to retire from full-contact play, primarily because I've had my bell rung a lot and want to preserve the few working brain cells I may have left. But I still watch the team play and hang out with the gang at parties, concerts, festivals, bars and, these days, microbreweries. And come the spring and summer months, I still play beach rugby, which is one of my favorite activities in life.

We started doing it thirty-some years ago, on a wide strip of scenic beach in front of what used to be a Howard Johnson's hotel. Ownership of the beachside resort has changed through the decades, but we're still meeting there every Thursday evening from April to October. We play a two-hand touch version of the game (tackle below the tide line) with no ref. Rules are loosely enforced, though often hotly debated, with whoever having possession of the ball at the time usually getting his, or her, way.

Teams are randomly selected amongst an assortment of old boys, current club players, gals from the women's team, and kids from local youth programs. We play till dark then gather at the hotel tiki bar, where we sit for hours drinking beer, having a bite to eat and telling lies. I'm not sure I can express the feeling you get from the combination of exercise, camaraderie and beer, all set in a slice of tropical paradise. With a briny breeze rustling palms, the moon rising over the sea and good cheer filling the air, we'll often look at each other and just smile, knowing that it *really* doesn't get much better than this.

Scientific studies show that this kind of fellowship improves several biomarkers of health, including blood pressure, body mass and inflammation. It also decreases risk of dementia and overall mortality.

"One's social life matters above and beyond what we already know about the 'quick fixes' of diet and exercise on health," says Yang Claire Yang, a sociologist at the University of North Carolina, Chapel Hill, who studies the physiological effects of social ties.

Of course, it's not necessary to take up rugby to find social connections. But if you can connect with folks who share some of the same interests through churches, clubs, volunteer work and the like, it will help your health and longevity.

Earthing

Despite all of the effort I expend playing touch rugby on a soft sandy beach, chasing around a bunch of really fit and/or young people, I always feel incredibly energized afterwards. Maybe it's due to all of those feel-good endorphins flooding my system from the exercise, camaraderie and craft beer. But it also may be at least partially due to Earthing.

Earthing, also called Grounding, is the idea that our planet's electro-magnetic energy can provide numerous health benefits to the human body if we actually come into contact with it more frequently. That means without rubber, plastic or other non-conductible materials coming between the planet's surface and us. Earthing was discovered by a retired cable TV pioneer named Clint Ober. Knowing that grounding TV cables helped prevent static in reception, he theorized it can do the same thing for people. The concept is that we can pick up electrons from the negatively-charged Earth to neutralize the positive-charged free radicals that wreak havoc inside the body by causing inflammation and the host of health woes that accompany it. And all you really have to do is walk around in footwear with natural soles that let through electrons from the earth or, better yet, go barefoot.

"Before 1960, when people stopped wearing leather-soled shoes, doctors mostly treated patients for injury or contagious disease," Ober told me for a story I did about Earthing. "Now, a lot of problems stem from chronic inflammation."

While it may sound bizarre, scientists are saying that the cable TV guy is onto something.

"Direct contact with the ground allows you to receive an energy infusion, compliments of Mother Earth," proclaims board-certified cardiologist Dr. Stephen Sinatra, Ober's co-author of the book *Earthing: The Most Important Health Discovery Ever!* "It can restore and stabilize the bioelectrical circuitry that governs your physiology and organs, harmonize your basic biological rhythms, boost self-healing mechanisms, reduce inflammation and pain, and improve your sleep and feeling of calmness."

Ober claims it helped him sleep better and get off meds for chronic pain. And a comprehensive review of nine Earthing studies concludes: "The research supports the concept that grounding the human body may be an essential element in the health equation along with sunshine, clean air and water, nutritious food, and physical activity."

Ober recommends Earthing forty-five minutes a day, walking barefoot on grass, rock or any other natural surface. The beach may be the best, he adds, because moisture, especially from salty seawater, improves conductivity.

"It's simple, yet so important," he says. "And it's free."

I think about old Clint every time I play beach rugby. There's little doubt I feel energized and sleep well those nights. And I'm now more apt to go barefoot in the yard. It can't hurt (unless I step on a rusty nail or into iguana shit), and it may help me to stay healthier through no cost or effort. Not sure you can beat that, especially if it works.

Stealth Health Problems

We've already covered a lot of material in this chapter with very little talk about beer. But to really enjoy the sudsy stuff, and life in general, you have to feel well. The body is such an incredible, self-healing piece of work, we tend to take our health for granted until something goes wrong. Then, nothing else really matters until we feel better, at which point we begin taking our health for granted again. We can only break the cycle by being proactive and paying attention to our body's needs before something goes wrong, and thus prevent problems.

Of course, no matter how well we coddle our bodies, shit happens. Many times, we go to a doc who can easily diagnose the problem (for example, gonorrhea) and prescribe some kind of treatment (a shot of penicillin in the butt and lecture about the use of condoms). But it seems with more and more frequency, the doc just scratches his or her head, and even after running a bunch of tests has trouble pinpointing the problem. Often, the symptoms - things like fatigue, diarrhea, joint pain, headaches, rashes and nausea – are common to many ailments.

During my time as a health writer, I've come across a handful of problems that easily fly under the radar. So if you're not feeling up to par and your doctor isn't sure why, check for these things:

Mold: If you have water stains in your home, school or workplace, chances are you're being exposed to toxic mold spores. The spores have been linked to a variety of ailments, including chronic fatigue, autoimmune disorders, digestive problems, hormonal disruptions, breathing trouble and neurological issues. Some people are genetically predisposed to be more sensitive to mold than others. A special urine test can detect the spores' toxins. Treatment consists of cleaning up the mold in the building and taking detoxifiers, such as the antioxidant glutathione and bentonite clay.

Leaky gut: Normally, intestinal tissue only lets small beneficial particles into the bloodstream, but malfunctions of gateways called intestinal tight junctions allow larger, potentially damaging things such as microbes and toxins to pass through. The body reacts by launching an inflammatory response, which can spark a variety of ailments and symptoms. Treatment consists of an anti-inflammatory, gluten-free diet, probiotics, digestive enzymes and omega-3 fatty acids, all of which support the integrity of intestinal tight junctions.

Parasites: Protozoan parasites are single-cell organisms that can cause diarrhea and other digestive problems. If they breach the intestinal tract and enter the bloodstream, they can affect organs, including the heart and brain. Worm parasites, called helminths, also affect the intestinal tract. And their excrement can trigger inflammatory reactions throughout the body, resulting in a variety of symptoms. Parasites are generally detected through stool samples and treated with prescription drugs.

Candida: Overgrowth of this yeast crowds out good gut flora and releases toxins that can cause chronic fatigue, mood swings, digestive problems, sinus infections, brain fog, hormonal imbalances, allergies, headaches, and the list goes on. High sugar consumption and antibiotics are two common triggers of candida overgrowth, which is diagnosed through a specialized stool test. Treatments include diet change, antifungal medication, probiotics and herbal therapies.

Lyme disease: Caused by tick-borne bacteria, Lyme disease is called The Great Imitator because symptoms can mirror so many other things, such as flu, arthritis, chronic fatigue, fibromyalgia, multiple sclerosis and Alzheimer's. The telltale sign is a bull's-eye rash around the tick bite, but not every victim gets it. The insidious disease can be particularly hard to both diagnose and treat because lab tests are unreliable, and although the bacteria can usually be killed if treated early with antibiotics, some bacteria may settle in a resistant, dormant form that can become activated months or even years later. While Lyme is mostly prevalent in the Northeast (it was discovered in Lyme, Connecticut), cases have now been identified in all fifty states.

Sleep apnea: We've already discussed the importance of sleep, and many beer-drinkers are totally unaware that they're even having a problem beyond a little snoring. But sawing wood is a classic symptom of obstructive sleep apnea (OSA), in which air flow to the lungs is periodically cut off. It comes back soon, so people with OSA typically don't wake up. But it's disruptive enough to keep them from getting into restorative states of sleep and causing a lot of health problems. Diagnosis involves at-home or sleep lab testing, and treatment consists of a CPAP mask that creates a pressurized airflow to keep airways open, or surgery to clear the obstruction.

Heavy metals: If you eat, drink, bathe and/or breathe, you are contaminated with at least trace levels of toxic heavy metals. Lead, mercury, cadmium and arsenic are the most prevalent in the environment, and our bodies, but there are a few dozen in all. Most of them have no biological role and cause trouble by various means, including oxidative stress and interference with enzyme reactions that allow cells to function properly. They can contribute significantly to heart disease, cancer, dementia, diabetes and just about every other chronic ailment you can name. Diagnosis is difficult because the destructive metal ions settle in tissue, making blood tests ineffective. The only proven way to reduce your heavy metal load is through chelation therapy, something I urge you to look into after recently completing a book called *The Chelation Revolution*. A series of infusions are the most effective way but also expensive and time-consuming. I use a suppository version that is more affordable and convenient. It's not pleasant to stick something up your butt every other night for months on end, but getting heart disease, cancer or Alzheimer's is sure to be a much bigger pain in the ass.

A Last Word About Lifestyle

Relax.

Stress is one of the most destructive forces to health. It basically speeds up the aging process and will ultimately lower your beer-drinking capacity. So keep in mind that very few things in life really matter in the long run. About 90 percent of the things we worry about never come to pass, and most of the stuff that does happen proves to be not as bad as we'd anticipated. The rest, to paraphrase Friedrich Nietzsche, either kills us or makes us stronger.

When I start getting upset about something, I ask myself: "Will this experience make for a funny story in a few hours, days, months or years?" Most often, the answer is, "Yes." And despite my distress, I can sometimes start laughing about it right then and there. It's said that laughter is the best medicine, and there's a lot of truth to that.

Chapter 9
Adventures in Homebrewing

After all of that stuff about diet, exercise and lifestyle, I think we need to spend a little time talking about beer, which we all love or we wouldn't be writing or reading this book. While I salivate over the seemingly endless variety of beer now available as close as your local supermarket (in most states), nothing beats drinking your own brew.

I often compare homebrew with homemade soup, which I also make. Unlike the store-bought versions, you can include what you want to most please your own taste buds. You also know exactly what is going into them, leaving out preservatives and other crap you see on labels that you can't pronounce. When reading ingredient labels, items you have to sound out syllable by syllable are probably things your body doesn't quite understand either.

But once again, I'm drifting from the point. Homebrew is awesome, not just because it tastes good but also because you made it yourself. I'm sure I'm biased, but I'd rather drink my own beer than just about anything else. In fact, I currently have sitting in my fridge a 16-ounce can of Arrogant Bastard Ale left over from before my January beer fast. For anyone unfamiliar with Arrogant Bastard – motto "You're not worthy" – it's a 7.2 percent ABV American strong ale with an attitude. "This is an aggressive beer," it states in the descriptive blurb on the back of the can. "You probably won't like it. It is quite doubtful you have the taste or sophistication to be able to appreciate a beer of this quality and depth." It backs up those words with a hoppy intensity that leaves its beady, toasted caramel malt backbone bravely clawing for parity and still falling a little bit short. Meanwhile, a note on the top rim of the can smugly suggests: "Drink fresh, numbskull."

Arrogant Bastard, created by the hop-heads at Stone Brewing in Escondido, California, is undoubtedly one of my favorite beers. So why, you may ask, has it been sitting on the top shelf of my refrigerator for over a month, especially when you have to be a numbskull not to drink it sooner than later? Well, it just so happens I had a batch of homebrew – two cases worth – waiting for me when I broke my beer fast on Groundhog Day. And every time I went into the fridge to grab a beer, I'd see the Bastard lurking in the back with his disdainful, I-dare-you-to-drink-me scowl, and I still consistently chose one of my own. Part of the reason is the flavor, which I see as being more balanced than the unrepentantly unbalanced Bastard, and part of the reason is my own ego and, yes, arrogance. Now down to my last three bottles of homebrew, I will be cracking open the Bastard soon and relish his "liquid arrogance" with every sip.

So, if you like beer enough to have read this far in the book, you probably should start brewing your own, if you haven't already. But don't expect to be challenging the Bastard right out of the blocks. There is a learning curve, and you can glean lot from my mistakes.

How NOT to Brew Beer

The first time I brewed up a pot of beer, my then teen son Glen and then family dog Lucky both kept their distance - and for good reason. Although the process of turning water, malt, hops and yeast into fine ale is not exactly rocket science, I was squawking and cursing up a storm at my own ineptitude.

"I wish to hell Nora had just given me a gift certificate to Total Wine!" I screamed to no one in particular after the burner blew out for the umpteenth time and I scorched my forearm on the brew pot yet again while trying to relight it.

Of course, Nora is my wife, and she had thoughtfully shelled out $125 to buy me a "deluxe" beer-brewing kit from the now defunct BX Beer Depot for the holidays. And Total Wine is the liquor superstore with a seemingly limitless assortment of delicious craft beers that you only need a fridge and bottle opener (or a strong set of teeth) to enjoy.

I don't recall all the problems I ran into during my maiden brew, but there were quite a few, and I was sure I'd screwed up what should have been a full-bodied, delightfully hopped India Pale Ale. One thing I know I did wrong was not account for the water boil-off. So I ended up with three-plus gallons of wort instead of five. Then, the gloppy, brown sludge that developed in the fermenter looked more like something you'd see flowing out of a latrine than beer tap. Wondering if I should replace the missing water, I called an expert at BX Beer Depot.

"Might be a little heavy," the expert said. "But don't add water during or after fermentation or it could end up tasting worse than a Coors Light clone."

The glop in the fermenter eventually cleared up pretty well, but I remained convinced I'd ruined the batch, and blown about $50 in supplies in the process. Still, I went to the trouble of bottling the brew. Then I anxiously waited a week or so for it to carbonate, chilled down a few bottles and popped the first one. It wasn't half-bad. After a couple, it was tasting pretty darn good. And it packed a punch, quickly washing away all the pains of beer-birth. By the silty bottom of my third bottle, I was already planning my next brew. But I was destined to encounter a few pitfalls, like…

Exploding Beer

Cleanliness is next to godliness when it comes to brewing, surprising since man first started making beer at the tail end of the Stone Age, when things were a lot dirtier than they are now. These days, everyone stresses that it is of upmost importance to make sure all of your brewing equipment is properly sanitized. Otherwise, your beer can get moldy or, worse, catch a bacterial infection. I had one batch develop a mold that spread across the surface of the beer during the second stage of its fermentation. My BX Beer Depot expert suggested I dump it, sanitize my equipment and try again. Not overly happy with that answer, I turned to homebrewing forums on the internet, asked the question and got several replies indicating I could simply siphon out the beer and leave the mold in the fermenter. One exception was a guy who said I'd no doubt ruined the batch and should send it to him for "evaluation." I decided to evaluate it myself, and the beer actually turned out excellent. I survived drinking it with no apparent ill effects, other than a few mushrooms growing out of my ears.

Bacterial infections are not so harmless. Well, actually, they are quite harmless to the human body when imbibed, but offensive to the nose and taste buds. I realized that my batch of White House Honey Brown Ale had been compromised while watching TV in bed one night. There was a "pop" in our home office (where my stash of freshly bottled ale was stored), and it turned out to one of the bottles exploding, spraying sticky honey brown ale all over the room. I immediately removed the two cases from the house, where they sat peacefully overnight then festered in the Florida heat the following day while I was at work.

Upon arriving home, I carried one case towards our detached laundry room, with intentions of popping the infected bottles and dumping them down a sink drain. But as I neared the laundry room, a bottle exploded. It broke at the base of the neck, and the capped end took off like an Atlas rocket, glancing off the side of my head before soaring over a six-foot fence into the neighbor's yard.

I then donned protective glasses, a long-sleeved shirt and gardening gloves, and cautiously proceeded to pop each of the forty-six remaining bottles, one-by-one, and pour them down the drain while emitting a fairly continuous stream of bad words. Needless to say, my son and the dog both kept their distance that afternoon, and by the end of the beer-shed, I had to hose out the laundry room.

So I never got a chance to taste the White House Honey Brown Ale, a recipe that was apparently enjoyed by then President Obama, who was gracious enough to share it with the world. I still have no idea how it got so badly infected, but even though I'm a Democrat, I'm not above blaming Obama.

That was the only one of many batches I've made that's blown up. Typically, you can prevent bacterial infections by using one of several types of sanitizers on the market. I prefer an iodine-based liquid concentrate, which is easy, cheap, effective and all you really need, so long so you don't involve the government.

Overflows

While some people brew beer in their kitchen, I highly recommend doing it outdoors on a propane burner, unless you think you may enjoy cleaning sticky wort residue from the deepest crevices in and around your stove area. Actually, the extract brewing process is pretty simple. First, you heat up three gallons of water to 150 degrees or so, turn off the flame and let a muslin sack with about a pound of crushed specialty grains steep for a half-hour, or long enough to play a game or two of horseshoes.

Then you remove the muslin sack from the now tea-colored water and compost or discard it (unless like me you save it for a neighbor with a pot-bellied pig named Mabel, who loves to eat the steeped grain). Bring the water to a boil, then add several pounds of malt extract, periodically sprinkle in a few ounces of hops for bittering, flavor and aroma, and boil it for about an hour. Once the wort is done, you add enough chilled water to bring it up to the five-gallon mark, and cool it down to about seventy-five degrees before pouring it into a fermenter, which looks like the kind of water bottle you see atop the water coolers at work where everyone is supposed to gather around to talk about current events or the boss and his secretary. You shake it up to aerate it, then add yeast, the magical-but-heat sensitive fungi that eats the sugars in the malt and converts them into alcohol and carbon dioxide.

But no matter how big your brew pot, at some point you are sure to experience an overflow. As the sugary malt boils, it can suddenly foam up and breach the lip of the brew pot, usually when you are momentarily distracted by a phone call, a late-arriving guest to your brew party or the dog choking on a chicken bone. The remedy is easy enough: kill the flame momentarily. But I can only imagine what a mess this would be in the kitchen, as opposed to outside, where the dog will lick up the spilt wort once he finishes spitting up or ingesting the chicken bone.

The ER

Exploding bottles aside, home beer brewing is normally a fairly safe hobby. Still, I once experienced a medical emergency during the beer chilling stage of the operation. Instead of spending about $70 on an immersion wort chiller (copper or stainless steel tubing that you run hose-water through), I'd freeze a one-gallon jug of spring water, sanitize it by dunking it in my iodine solution, then carefully cut the plastic all the way around with a sanitized blade to free the block of ice before dumping it in the wort.

For more than three years, this method worked fine, even though combining a razor-sharp blade with a slippery object and an afternoon of beer-drinking seemed inherently catastrophic. One Sunday afternoon, as I cut off the plastic and chatted with pals, the blade slipped and encountered my wrist. It took two hours, six stiches and a $200 emergency room co-pay to fix, so I now use a wort chiller.

But I did finish up that batch. And you know what? It was bloody good beer.

A Brew For Two

I'm sure that more arrogant homebrewers than I grimace at the fact that, after several years, I still do extract brewing as opposed to whole grain, which is cheaper as far as ingredients go and offers a much wider variety of options. In the whole grain process, you have to mash and sparge several pounds of crushed grains before boiling, which takes a couple of hours and more equipment. With extract, the grains have already been processed into a syrup or powder. So it's easier, less time consuming, and there's a pretty wide range of malts to choose from and/or combine.

Lately, I've been trying to develop a beer that my wife and I both like. It's tough because she historically doesn't like hoppy beers and I do. She clearly lacks the taste and sophistication of an Arrogant Bastard aficionado and has a childish habit of crinkling her nose and handing a beer like that back to me, which is kind of good because, well, there's more for me.

But I do like to share things with my wife, so I made it a mission to brew something we could both enjoy. After a few failures, I finally created a recipe that worked. The key is in the bittering hops, which needed to be fairly robust but not overpowering. I found one that straddled the line in a strain called Calypso, which happens to be the name of the soccer team Nora used to play with in New Orleans. The first time I offered her a sip, she took one, said, "Not bad," and kept the bottle. Then the most amazing thing happened. My wife, who frowns on beer at a temperature anywhere above 33 degrees F, set it down momentarily to attend to a leaning tomato plant in the garden, got distracted by other agrarian emergencies, and let the beer get warm (it doesn't take long in South Florida). Knowing how disgruntled I get when someone wastes one of my homebrews, she chanced a sip anyway and looked almost startled as she proclaimed: "This tastes just as good warm, maybe even better."

So now we have a beer we can drink together, which is kind of good because we have something else to bond over but also kind of bad because, well, there's less for me.

Brew Parties

Like sex, brewing is more fun when you do it with others. Invite friends to come over to help, learn how to brew or just sit around drinking beer, talking about sports, cars, beer or other important topics and maybe squeezing in a few games of cards, backgammon or horseshoes. Meanwhile, if your significant other is anything like Nora, she will probably feed you all, in part because she can't just sit around and do nothing on account of her being a woman. If you ask each guest to bring some kind of relatively exotic ale, everyone will get a chance to taste-test a variety of them, and any leftovers will generally end up in your fridge. One of the nicest things about brewing is that you really don't have to do much, which leaves plenty of time to do what guys do best – nothing in particular. And if you're a female brewer, it offers plenty of time for what you do best - accomplish something else.

Chapter 10
The Demon Alcohol

Well, we've put this off for about as long as we can but must finally address the elephant in the taproom. As I have mentioned earlier, the one really unhealthy thing about beer is the alcohol. And for many of us, indications of the Demon's destructive powers were pretty evident from our earliest experiences with him.

Do you remember the first time you got drunk?

Mine was a doozy. It was the summer of 1969. I was almost sixteen and visiting one of my best friends in Barnegat Light on the Jersey shore. Todd's family had a small house there and, as I recall, another pal, Rob, and I took a train from the Philly area to Atlantic City, where Todd's mom or dad picked us up for a short ride up the coast. I don't remember much of anything we did, other than going to a party one night at an apartment. It was packed with older kids. Music was blaring and bottles were being passed around. I latched onto some Boone's Farm Apple Wine, which tasted a lot like apple juice. But with every swig I felt happier and happier. I was normally shy, especially around girls. But suddenly I found talking to them very easy, and a few seemed to be downright charmed by this cute little runt telling them how beautiful they were. One blue-eyed brunette took a fancy to me, but more like a big sister than anything else.

"You better watch out how much you drink," she warned.

I no doubt smiled stupidly and said something like, "No problem. I feel great. Have I told you how beautiful you are?"

In fact, it was just about the best feeling in the world, until Rob and I got back to Todd's home. At the party, I'd followed up the Boone's Farm with some other fruity wine and maybe a sugary cocktail or two, and when I fell into bed, everything went spinning round and round, including the contents of my stomach, which soon erupted out onto the concrete floor by my bed. Todd, who had not been with Rob and me at the party, was a good sport in helping me clean up the mess and, come morning, I awoke with a hangover so severe it permanently etched itself into my memory bank. All of the fluids seemed to have been drained from my body. My lips were cracked, and throat parched, as if I'd been lost in the desert with no water for days. The back of my eyelids felt like sandpaper, my body ached and my head pounded like kettle drums. Todd's family was eating a hearty breakfast and seemed amused by my condition. Nausea welled at the sight and smell of the food. I could barely force a few sips of water past my dry lips without feeling an urge to puke again.

Rob wasn't in much better shape, but we still had to somehow make our way back home that day. For some reason, we hitchhiked rather than taking public transport, and it was torturous. I'm not sure which was worse, waiting in the hot summer sun for rides or bouncing around in the back seat of various vehicles. It was the worst I'd ever felt, and that was saying a lot since the previous year I'd broken my femur in a car accident and spent ten weeks in traction and ten more in assorted casts. I do remember looking at Rob and proclaiming: "I. Will. Never. Drink. Again."

The driver found this amusing (hangovers are inherently amusing to everyone who isn't hungover) and informed me that everyone says the same thing but winds up getting drunk again at some point.

All I could think was, "Boy, is he ever wrong. Nothing is worth this."

The Demon's Lure

Obviously, the driver was right. The first killer hangover rarely drives people into a lifetime of abstinence. Typically, it is a rite of passage into adulthood, where the Demon lies in wait. He's a con man, pretending to be your pal and convincing you that you can do anything: win that game, get that job, charm that gal, put your hand on that dartboard and see if your friend can throw a dart between your fingers…

In small doses, the Demon can be a positive influence in your life, and even in your body. But too much of him leaves you with a dart hole in your finger, and it gets worse from there.

Dealing with the Demon is a matter of balance. There's a fine line between enjoying his charms and falling into his clutches. You are King, or Queen, and he is the court jester. When those roles start to reverse, you have to banish him for a while - an hour, day, week, month, year, or more. Whatever it takes to keep you the master.

Here's the problem if you don't.

For starters, too much alcohol can shrink the brain, so you have less gray matter to deal with things like work, play, social interactions and pretty much everything else short of binge-watching *The Walking Dead*. And along with those atrophied cells go some of your memory, especially short-term, which is why you may forget exactly how you pissed off your boss at the office Christmas party after OD-ing on the eggnog.

Too much alcohol weakens the heart muscle and can mess with its rhythm, two very important factors in doing anything, including staying alive. It can also raise blood pressure, which damages the heart's blood vessels. And anything that compromises the heart is likely to reduce its ability to effectively supply blood to all other parts of the body, which can compromise pretty much all of you.

Too much alcohol really fucks with your liver, perhaps the hardest working organ in the body. One of its many functions is to filter toxins, like alcohol, from the blood and metabolize them for elimination. It takes about one hour for the liver to process the amount of alcohol in a standard drink, and if you drink faster than that, the extra alcohol hangs out waiting, raising your blood alcohol content (BAC) to the point where you may need to Uber home. Too much overload over a course of time will eventually start damaging the liver tissue, first making it fatty (fatty liver disease), then scarred (cirrhosis), then dead, along with the rest of your body (rigor mortis).

Brain, heart and liver are the Big Three, and dysfunction in any of them can suck the joy out of life. Too much alcohol also irritates the digestive tract, alters pancreatic function, damages kidneys, weakens immunity, throws hormones out of whack and disrupts sleep, among other things. Apart from direct hits to the body, too much alcohol increases harm through accident, domestic abuse, gunshot wounds, road rage and, yes, seeing if your friend can throw a dart between your fingers (something Jose Cuervo once convinced a pal of mine to try, with expected results).

One takeaway from all this is to at least try not to outdrink your liver's capacity to process the alcohol. That works out to one 12-ounce can of 5 percent ABV Budweiser per hour, as opposed to a pint of 8 percent ABV Pliny the Elder, which would take the liver closer to two hours. Limiting yourself like that can be hard to do in a party situation, especially after a rugby game. But you should at least be aware of how your body works and be willing to give it a break between brews. I try to alternate beer with water, which not only decreases my alcohol consumption but also helps to keep me hydrated. And if you favor higher gravity beers, such as our elder friend Pliny, you may want to pepper in some lower-alcohol brews, such as All Day IPA from Grand Rapids, Michigan-based Founders brewery. It weighs in at just 4.7 percent ABV but has the flavor of a much stronger ale. "Session" beers like All Day IPA are an easy and satisfying swap.

Another great tip is to not drink on an empty stomach. We all like to eat, so this shouldn't be too taxing. Pretty much any type of food will slow down the absorption of alcohol, making it easier for your liver to keep up with the demand. But experts recommend foods high in healthy fats and lean protein.

Fighting Back

So the Demon is out to get you, but you can fight back. Unlike regular warfare, where the bigger the gun, or nuclear weapon, the better, in this war you have to think small. The real damage alcohol inflicts on your body is carried out on a cellular level. So that is the ultimate battlefield. And while you can't generate an impenetrable force field to protect yourself, you may be able to at least blunt the Demon's relentless attack.

To explain all of this may get a bit technical (boring), but some beer drinkers, like me, are inherently curious about the way things work. Others can skip through it, but should at least take note of some of the supplements (conveniently highlighted in **boldface**) they can take to reduce the impact of alcohol on the body.

Basically, the Demon drains cells of certain nutrients, which could otherwise be utilized to help regulate metabolism, fight pathogens (viruses, bacteria and other invaders), dispose of waste, repair DNA and manage other vital functions. Fewer nutrients mean less efficient processing of all this stuff, which can lead to fatigue, disease, inflammation and other dysfunction, including the most immediate, the hangover, which we will discuss separately later on.

Alcohol can also lead to weight gain. That's because the liver breaks it down into a toxin called acetaldehyde, which is then mostly converted into acetate, a calorie-dense energy source that the body will burn off before carbohydrates. That means the calories you get from the alcohol in beer will be used before the calories you get from the loaded nachos and stuffed potato skins. And the carbs that don't get burned end up as fat, producing weight gain.

The process of alcohol metabolism depletes many nutrients including:

- **Nicotinamide adenine dinucleotide (NAD).** This coenzyme is in all living things and has a central role in biological functions. Levels naturally go down as we age, and drinking exacerbates that problem. While you can't take NAD directly in pill form, there two related supplements called **nicotinamide riboside** and **nicotinamide mononucleotide** that help the body produce more NAD.
- **N-acetylcysteine (NAC).** This amino acid binds with acetaldehyde, reducing alcohol toxicity. It is an especially efficient detoxifier when combined with **vitamin C**.
- **Glutathione.** An important detoxifying agent and antioxidant, glutathione is naturally produced by the body and is most highly concentrated in the liver. But the Demon sops it up, which can lead to liver cell damage and systemic oxidative stress.
- **B-complex vitamins.** Alcohol inhibits the absorption of these vitamins, with thiamine (B1) the most affected.
- **Vitamin E.** Even moderate alcohol consumption depletes the body's reserves of this antioxidant, and studies show that replenishing it can protect you against alcohol-related oxidative stress and inflammation.

- **Selenium.** This trace mineral, which is an important cog in the antioxidant process, is another nutrient directly affected by alcohol.

Supplements for all of these nutrients are as close as your nearest pharmacy, health food store or internet connection. Other supplements that support alcohol-related depletion are:

- **Milk thistle.** Silymarin is the active ingredient in this prickly plant, and it helps to repair liver cells, fight inflammation and prevent the depletion of glutathione.
- **Clove bud extract.** A scientific study found that a single 250 mg dose of clove bud extract taken before drinking led to lower blood alcohol and acetaldehyde concentrations, less depletion of detoxification enzymes, and less severe hangover symptoms than a control group.
- **Grape Seed Extract.** Grape seeds and skins are a rich source of polyphenolic compounds that neutralize tissue-damaging free radicals associated with alcohol consumption.
- **Probiotics.** The Demon wreaks havoc on your microbiome. He feeds the bad bacteria in your gut, crowding out the good stuff. But probiotic supplements can help mitigate the damage.

I don't suggest you run out to your local health food store, or to the internet, to order all of these supplements, but you may want to try a few of them if you are a regular drinker. A high-quality B-complex supplement and milk thistle is a good start. Dietary supplement giant Life Extension also offers Anti-Alcohol capsules with what they describe as "broad-spectrum nutrients designed to combat free radicals, neutralize alcohol metabolites such as acetaldehyde, and support healthy liver function."

Beer Break

It's getting around to happy hour again, and today I have a special treat for us. It's a beer brewed using a recipe by Thomas Jefferson, the Founding Father who famously wrote, "We hold these truths to be self-evident that all beers are not created equal," in the Declaration of Brew-dependence, or something like that. When I first tasted this beer, from Philadelphia's own Yards Brewing Co., it was called Tavern Ale but has since been rechristened Jefferson's Golden Ale, even though it is more copper than gold in hue.

I first discovered Jefferson's brew on one of my family's annual trips to attend the Philadelphia Folk Festival. On the way from the airport to my brother Rick's house, we always stop in New Jersey to stock up on beer and other inebriants for the Fest because it's a lot cheaper there than in Pennsylvania, which apparently never got over being founded by Quaker teetotalers and wants you to pay more for your sinful drinking ways. I mostly buy stuff I can't get in Florida, and I was intrigued by Yards' Ales of the Revolution variety pack. It included Washington's Porter, Poor Richard's Spruce Ale (from Ben Franklin's recipe) and Jefferson's Tavern Ale, which was clearly the best of the lot.

Said to be brewed "employing honey, rye and wheat," it has a very distinct flavor that is initially sweet before the bitterness and 8 percent ABV booziness kick in. It's a sipping beer, which isn't really conducive to the Fest, where you tend to drink beer all day and through most of the night.

Still, I can't resist having a few, here and there between less potent brews and, of course, plenty of water.

Whenever a friend or relative from Philly comes to visit me in Florida and asks what they can bring, Tom Jefferson's ale is what I tell them. Unfortunately, it can't be transported in carry-ons, so I rarely get any. But on a recent trip here, Rick checked his bag and included a couple of bottles left over from the last Fest. I'd like to share one with you now to celebrate our Creator-endowed unalienable rights, which include life, liberty and the pursuit of good beer.

Dealing with Hangovers

Because we love beer so much, we sometimes love it too much. Often, it's not just the beer that will get you, but also the kamikazes, snifters of bourbon, frozen margaritas and other inebriants you may find impossible to resist in addition to the beer. In any case, the end result is not pleasant - a splitting headache, cotton mouth, queasy tummy and untimely demise of countless brain cells that you might actually miss in your Golden Years.

Almost as bad as the hangover is hearing about some of the home remedies that people swear by, such as drinking pickle brine or a "prairie oyster" (tomato juice, tabasco, Worcestershire sauce, salt, pepper and raw egg), or even putting slices of lemons under your arms (really). Pliny the Elder reputedly recommended munching a deep-fried canary, which the PETA people probably wouldn't be happy about today. The oldest known hangover remedy was written in Greek on papyrus and details how wearing a necklace made from the leaves of an Alexander laurel shrub will banish the "drunken headache." Good luck with that one. Others swear that all it takes to banish a hangover is to "have a nip of the hair of the dog that bit you," meaning to start drinking again.

I'm not sure if any of those things work or not. The only one I've tried is the last one, which I believe is why Bloody Marys were invented. Even if imbibing more alcohol may make you feel better, it's really just a temporary fix and will ultimately pile additional abuse on your poor, overworked liver and further deplete those vital nutrients your body needs to function properly.

Fortunately for all of us, I once did a story about Hangover Heaven, a Las Vegas-based service that uses intravenous-administered concoctions to cure hangovers. The business was conceived and operated by Dr. Jason Burke, a young anesthesiologist who found a way to make even more money than your average physician by appealing to people who don't want to waste any vacation time suffering from a bender when it could be better spent losing money at craps or watching Wayne Newton perform.

"With my treatment protocol, I can take you from a semi-conscious, porcelain-hugging, hit-by-a-truck hangover to feeling like you're ready to take on the world in less than forty-five minutes," boasts Burke. "I think this is a major development in medicine."

Burke considers himself the world's foremost authority on the hangover, evident by the fact he seems to be the only one in the world who calls it by its medical name, veisalgia. He also claims to have treated more cases of veisalgia than anyone else on the planet, and he doesn't seem too keen on the prairie oyster or fried canaries.

Burke busts the popular belief that the primary cause of a hangover is dehydration.

"Pro basketball players get dehydrated during a game, and they don't end up with headaches, nausea and other hangover symptoms," he explains. "The main causes are inflammation and oxidative stress. Processing alcohol creates free radicals, which basically cause cells to self-destruct."

And the older you are, the longer it takes to repair the damage.

"When you're twenty, you get over a hangover in a day," says Burke. "When you're thirty it may take a couple of days, and over forty it can take a week or more to fully get over it."

That is, unless you can afford one of Burke's IV Hangover Hydration Cures, which range from $199 for the "Salvation" option to $329 for the "Eternity." High rollers who are epically incapacitated can splash an extra $100 to be treated in their hotel room. The problem for most of us is that to take advantage of Burke's services, you have to not only have a wad of disposable cash but also be in Las Vegas. If you, or anyone you know, is a compounding pharmacist, you could whip up your own batch at home. The recipe includes the potent antioxidants glutathione and taurine along with magnesium, anti-inflammatory, anti-nausea and anti-heartburn medications, B vitamins and vitamin C, all delivered through an IV in a hydrating solution.

Of course, like a majority of medical problems, the most effective treatment for a hangover is prevention.

"The most important thing is to prepare before you start drinking," says Burke. "Give your body the tools it needs to best deal with the alcohol."

The first tip, as already mentioned, is to not drink on an empty stomach. Burke also suggests taking some supplements, such as his Hangover Prevention Pill.

"Hangovers are pretty complex conditions, causing headache, nausea, and overall misery, so multiple ingredients are needed," he notes. "Antioxidants include taurine, alpha lipoic acid, vitamins B, C and E, and milk thistle. Natural anti-inflammatories include curcumin, aloe and boswellia."

And whether or not you prepare yourself for a night of drinking, try not to just flop into bed at the end. Burke recommends drinking some water (not too much) and taking Advil to reduce inflammation. Make sure to avoid painkillers with acetaminophen, like Tylenol, because they can be tough on the liver and kidneys when combined with the Demon.

"The human body was not designed to drink alcohol," says Burke. "So take precautions. It's much easier to prevent a hangover than deal with it in the morning."

Chapter 11
Living Hoppily Ever After

This is it. The final chapter. It's a Wednesday evening, the clocks poised to spring forward this coming weekend and turn an hour of night back into day. I'm sipping a 7 percent ABV Redfish Red IPA from Flying Fish Brewing Company, of Somerdale, New Jersey, and starting to feel a little warm and fuzzy. With this book coming to an end, I must say that I will miss chatting with you about three of my favorite things: beer, health and myself.

I like Flying Fish beers, which are not only satisfying to the palate but also the purse, as a six-pack of Redfish longnecks can be had for $6.99 at Total Wine with a dollar-off coupon. This one happens to be part of a modestly priced variety 12-pack and includes a golden IPA, an abbey dubbel and a citra-hopped pale ale. All are tasty and pack a little punch. Flying Fish is one of my go-to breweries, where I know I won't be disappointed. Stone, Rogue, Dogfish Head, Boulevard, Ommegang, Sierra Nevada, Sam Adams and, of course my local favorite, Barrel of Monks, are some others, to name a few. And more and more continually pop up on the landscape. As far as I'm concerned, we're living in the Golden Age of Beer.

Coincidentally, since turning sixty-five in 2018, I am officially in my Golden Years. This is a time when things are supposed to slow down as we retire from work and mosey along a path of low resistance towards the sunset of our lives. Unfortunately, I kind of retired when I was young, traveling around a lot and not working much, so I will likely have to toil away writing until I die. That's no big deal since I would probably write anyway, because writing is part of my being.

A potentially more disrupting part of our Golden Years is the ever-increasing chance that they will be tarnished by health woes as our bodies slowly run out of juice. In a way, health is all about energy, where we get it from and how we process it. It powers the life force that runs our bodies, allowing us to think and move and drink beer. It also maintains our bodies, fixing broken parts or breaking down and recycling parts that are beyond repair.

This energy goes by many names - *Qi* to the Chinese, *Prana* to Hindus, *Ka* to ancient Egyptians and so on. Interestingly, Hippocrates, the Father of Modern Medicine, called it the Healing Power of Nature. Yet most modern-day doctors, who typically take some version of the Hippocratic Oath upon receiving their medical degrees, don't really pay it much mind when treating disease. Often, they scoff at therapists, such as chiropractors, acupuncturists and our beloved Dr. Corey, who do focus on using this life force to heal.

One of those doubting docs is a family friend who recently visited me in Florida. A seventy-year-old radiologist, his body has been deteriorating alarmingly over the past few years. He's had a hip replaced, and needs the other one done as well as both knees. His hair has fallen out, his ankles are chronically swollen, and his once trim, athletic body has a jelly belly that flops over his belt. Through the years, he's tried to fight off aging with a variety of pharmaceuticals and, at one point, human growth hormone. But they don't seem to be slowing his decline.

"God doesn't love you after you hit sixty-five," he grouses.

It's true in a way. We were designed to break down at some point to make way for new models of humans that are better adapted to survive. That's why, outside of a few rugby players, you don't see any Neanderthals walking around these days. It's the process of evolution, with God, or Mother Nature, or The Force, or whatever you want to call it constantly tinkering with all species. But to make room for the new, improved versions, you have to get rid of the old ones.

At least that's the way it's always been. We now have evolved to the point where we are starting to do a little tinkering ourselves. Technology has allowed us to better understand how our bodies work and why they break down. It seems to have less to do with God than chemistry, as imbalances in the substances needed to run our body processes disrupt our genetic programming and cause dysfunction. If we can somehow straighten out, or prevent, these chemical imbalances to keep our cells functioning the way they're supposed to, we can slow down or even stop the aging process. We may even be able to reverse it.

Researchers have recently dubbed the study of aging geroscience.

"Geroscience is kind of a reversal of the way biomedical research has been practiced," explains Matt Kaeberlein, a University of Washington researcher and co-director of the Dog Aging Project, a comprehensive study of longevity in man's best friend. "Instead of waiting for a disease to be diagnosed before treating it, we try to understand the biological mechanisms of aging that cause the diseases so we can find interventions that delay the onset or slow the progression of them. It's the ultimate preventative medicine."

Kaeberlein's research is designed to learn not only how to increase longevity in dogs, but also humans. Early results of the three-phase study suggest that the pharmaceutical drug rapamycin, primarily used today to treat certain kinds of cancers and as an anti-rejection therapy for transplant patients, may also trick the body into thinking it's not getting enough nutrients, so it goes into a preservation mode. The end result, he expects, will be a 15 percent increase in lifespan.

Nearly as impressive as his studies, Kaeberlein managed to wheedle some funding from the government, which is unusual for geroscientists.

"Moneywise, things are getting better," he says. "But geroscience is still woefully underfunded."

Stayin' Alive

Others are even more ambitious and are actually seeking immortality. Eternal life has always been the stuff of legends, not reality. But a growing number of people believe we are on the verge of dealing a serious blow to the funeral home business. Counterculture icon and LSD proponent Dr. Timothy Leary was the first one I heard about who proclaimed that immortality was achievable in his generation's lifetime. He happened to be dead wrong, at least in his case. In 1996, he left the earthly realm at age seventy-nine following a battle with prostate cancer. Ironically, that was well after the Moody Blues immortalized Leary in the 1968 song *Legend of the Mind,* including the lyrics: "Timothy Leary's dead…no, no, no, no…he's on the outside looking in." Despite Leary's untimely demise, other less astral planetary folks have jumped on the immortality bandwagon, including Bill Faloon.

Faloon is the co-founder and driving force behind the Life Extension Foundation, which has not only developed and sold a gazillion dietary supplements but has also sunk more than $100 million into longevity-associated scientific research. Faloon has endured a few run-ins with the FDA, but survived them all and is now regarded as something of a demi-god in some anti-aging circles. He says his fascination with immortality dates back to his childhood.

"When I was eight years old, my mother said I was going to die someday and there was nothing I could do about it," he recalls. "In that moment, and every single day of my life thereafter, I thought I'd have to try to find some way around this death issue."

So far, so good. At sixty-six, Faloon looks decades younger with thick dark hair and barely a wrinkle on his face. To fight off Father Time, he sticks to a low-calorie diet (something like 1,500 a day), stays inside a lot to avoid the damaging radiation of the sun, and probably drinks little, if any, beer. He also takes about twenty-five supplements a day and seems game to try just about anything that research suggests may improve longevity. That includes a few prescription medications, such as the diabetes drug metformin, and alternative and even experimental therapies. He credits infusions of the vital coenzyme NAD for helping him to overcome a potentially deadly genetic bone marrow condition, and he expresses high hopes for embryo stem cell therapy and young plasma transfusions, among other things. Still, he knows that the clock continues to tick, as his quest for immortality is a race against time.

"Through our Society for Age Reversal, I work with researchers from every major country and have a network of people seeking to end biological aging within next twelve years," he says. "Not everyone wants to live forever. But the prospect of living indefinitely means you can do everything you've always wanted to do because there is no upper limit age threshold."

While I respect Faloon's quest, I don't think that I'd want to live forever doing what he does. And I believe I speak for all beer-lovers, some of whom may not even stick to under 1,500 calories a day in beer. Another problem is that Faloon's longevity-boosting methods can be quite costly for someone who doesn't run a multimillion-dollar dietary supplement company. You could make a decent case for taking dozens of supplements a day, because they all have different vital nutrients, many of which are sorely lacking in most people's daily diets. But that could cost hundreds of dollars a month, if not more, and I doubt anyone would want to live forever in poverty.

A New Hope

But don't despair. There may be another way for you to have your beer and longevity, too. And that path has been forged by Dr. Sandra Kaufmann, the forty-nine-year-old chief of anesthesiology at Joe DiMaggio Children's Hospital in Hollywood, Florida. She's also a molecular biologist and rising star in the tight community of anti-aging proponents since the 2018 publication of her book, *The Kaufmann Protocol: Why We Age and How to Stop It.*

"One day in my forties, I'd had it with aging," she writes in the forward of her book. "I didn't want to look old, I didn't want to feel old, and I certainly didn't want to act old. In what has been called the most productive outcome of a mid-life crisis, I set out to overcome aging, but in a logical way. I began plowing through thousands and thousands of legitimate, scientific research papers to determine if there was anything of substance I could do to stave off the effects of time."

To her "gleeful shock," she found fourteen "molecular agents" that she believes can help stop Father Time in his tracks, or at least slow him down to a crawl. It all has to do with the health of cells, which she compares to tiny factories that need seven distinct things: an operating system (DNA), energy (mitochondria), work flow (metabolic pathways), maintenance (repair and recycling), security (immune system), workers (the cells themselves) and waste management (excretion). When things get fouled up in any of the departments, it can disrupt production. When cells don't produce, body functions decline. Just like old factories, old cells are more likely to experience problems, which lead to ailments of aging, such as cancer, Alzheimer's, arthritis, osteoporosis, heart disease and a passion for early bird dinners.

Kaufmann serves as her own guinea pig, and the results have been dramatic. An avid rock climber, she recently went on an expedition to the base camp of Mount Everest. As she hiked ever higher, others in the group were amazed at how she didn't even seem to be breathing hard. One of the mountaineers, who was on his way to actually scale the world's highest peak, noted what great shape she was in and asked what she'd done to train for the trek.

"I took a shitload of astragalus," she replied.

Astragalus is a medicinal herb that triggers red blood cell production to help optimize oxygen absorption, which comes in handy during high-altitude expeditions. It is also proven to slow telomere loss and is one of the fourteen substances included in Kaufmann's protocol.

I met Kaufmann through one of my rugby pals, who is also a climber.

"When we were on climbing trips," he told me, "Sandy would keep talking about telomeres and mitochondria and all of these other things I'd never heard of, and I told her you have to talk to my friend Gary because he's a health writer and into all of that stuff, too."

It's been a symbiotic relationship, as I've raked in some nice paychecks writing stories about her for several publications (including *Life Extension* magazine), and the publicity has helped her to sell books and gain a solid foothold with the anti-aging crowd. My wife and I have also started following her protocol, taking five of the substances that, together, support all seven cellular needs at a price even a freelance writer can afford. She's dubbed the five the "PANACEA," which is a stretch as an acronym for the substances but sums up the impact. The most noticeable effect is more energy, which says a lot. If my body has more energy to bike harder and do more push-ups, you've got to figure it has more energy to maintain and heal itself.

Kaufmann has graciously offered to let me share her PANACEA with you, but you really should also buy her book, which is "dedicated to all the mice and rats that have given up their lives to help the rest of us live better and longer."

All of these things are affordable and readily available. I'm not going to recommend any specific brands, but you need to do some research because the supplement industry is rife with substandard products. Cheap store brands and generics often contain contaminated ingredients and fillers, and can even be mislabeled. Look for companies that adhere to Good Manufacturing Practice (GMP) regulations and are certified by third-party watchdogs such as NSF International or US Pharmacopeia (USP).

Pterostilbene: Like its better-known cousin resveratrol, this fat-soluble plant polyphenol supports all seven categories of cell health. It's one of the few substances that activate sirtuins, a family of proteins that regulate the body's metabolic pathways and play a vital role in the function of mitochondria, the generators that power cells. Resveratrol has similar benefits, but pterostilbene is better absorbed by the body and stays active in the bloodstream much longer.

Astaxanthin: A super-potent antioxidant, this carotenoid is most abundant in a common algae and has remarkable powers to fight free radicals, oxidative stress and inflammation. Due to its ability to permeate both cell and mitochondrial membranes, it has more than fifty times the antioxidant capability of vitamin C and is particularly effective in supporting a cell's energy generation and immunity.

Nicotinamide riboside/mononucleotide: As you may recall from the chapter on alcohol, these nicotinamide supplements are a precursor that the body easily converts into the coenzyme NAD. The Demon is a huge drain on our diminishing production of NAD, which is vital for energy generation. It also plays pivotal roles in DNA repair and sirtuin function.

Curcumin: A compound found in the curry spice turmeric, curcumin supports five of the seven categories of cell health. One if its strengths is in the waste management department, where it can reduce the amount of lipofuscin, a metabolism byproduct that accumulates in cells, especially long-living ones like those in the brain. But you can't eat enough turmeric to reap its benefits. Since curcumin is hard for the body to process, look for a product with high bio-availability.

Carnosine: This dipeptide is manufactured in muscles from amino acids we get through eating animal products. Although it offers support for telomeres (the protective caps on genes) and is a great free radical scavenger, carnosine is most valuable for removing the destructive byproducts created when we burn glucose for energy. They're called advanced glycogen end products (AGEs), and they gum up the works. Among other things, AGEs prevent proteins from doing their jobs and cause collagen to break down, leading to stiff blood vessels, saggy skin and other hallmarks of aging. "Carnosine is magic," says

Kaufmann. "If you put old cells in a bath of carnosine, they become youthful again."

Last Thoughts

Since Dolly Neuman first gave me a Miller High Life on a boat in Maryland a half-century ago, my beer consumption has been an ongoing evolution. In my early drinking years, there wasn't much of a selection. Schlitz and Pabst Blue Ribbon were about as good as it got. Coors, which was only distributed out West, had a mystique that made it desirable back East, until you tasted it. But my beer world changed when I tried pricy Löwenbräu, a German bier that cost about double the American varieties, but was worth it (at least until Miller acquired the North American rights and began brewing it domestically). Löwenbräu was the first beer I considered a real treat, and it opened the door to other European brands, like Heineken, Carlsberg (especially the Elephant Malt), Beck's, creamy black Guinness stout and the British pale ale Bass.

In the early 1990s, I was a teaching assistant in Florida International University's Master of Fine Arts Creative Writing program in North Miami. One term, I had a late afternoon Shakespeare comedy class and taught an evening freshman comp course. Between the two, I sometimes treated myself to a meal at the nearby Gourmet Diner, which was basically an old-fashioned aluminum-sided diner that had been converted into what I assumed to be a French restaurant. On an evening when things were uncharacteristically slow, the proprietor waited on me. He was actually Belgian and grimaced when I ordered a Heineken.

"You want to try something really good?" he asked, and brought me a Belgian tripel that rocked my world. (I'm sure it came from a brewery similar in name to Germany's Mönchshof, but can find no trace of it or that Mönchshof ever produced a tripel.) The complexity of flavors and mule-like kick left me with an undying affinity for Belgian brews. The problem back then was that when I finally tracked down a six-pack of the stuff on the liquor store side of my local Big Daddy's bar, it was $12, way beyond the paygrade of a graduate student with a baby on the way.

My beer evolution splintered in many directions with the rise of the craft brewing industry in the new millennium, and my exposure to it through the late Case & Keg bottle shop. There is now an embarrassingly rich selection of awesome brews, and I don't want to stop boldly exploring this ever-expanding new frontier.

But to do so, I must make some sacrifices to preserve my health. That means rousing myself at daybreak to get some regular exercise, eating sensibly most of the time, fasting one day a week and, yes, limiting my beer consumption, including a torturous month-long beer fast.

I could quite easily drink myself to death and leave this world with a smile on my face. But I'd rather keep drinking and smiling while alive for as long as I can, because there's always a new beer to taste and new batch to brew, and I don't want to miss any of it.

Final Beer Break

I now have before me a freshly poured glass of Rexx, an imperial red ale aged in bourbon barrels from Boston-based Clown Shoes Beer. I'd never heard of it before my last visit to Total Wine, but the T-Rex dinosaur clad in clown shoes on the label of the bomber bottle caught my eye, and I've always been a sucker for red ale, not to mention a 10 percent ABV. Still, at $13.99 I was going to pass on it because some leftover bombers of Santa's Reserve – one of my favorite brews in any season – were now, in mid-March, on sale for a scant $4.99.

"Just get it," my lovely wife Nora urged.

I wavered. "But I can get nearly three bottles of Santa's Reserve for one Rexx," I said.

Nora sighed. We'd recently gotten the sad news of a friend who'd died just weeks after retiring.

"Get them all," she said. "Let's enjoy life while we can."

So I did, and as the first sip passes my lips and swirls around my palette, the near-syrupy taste is a bit overwhelming until the alcohol and bourbon barrel-aged nuance bring it back from the edge. There is little hop presence to interfere with the flavors of caramel, molasses and tart fruit of the full-bodied malt. It's a little sweet for my hop-tempered taste buds, but seems to get better with each sip, as good beers will do.

As I finish the first glass, the stress from another workday of life during the rapid decline of Western civilization fades away. I will have the second glass out by Stella's turtle pen, so I'll bid farewell to you now with wishes for good health, good beer, and warm and fuzzy feelings for many years to come.

Appendix I
Healthy Soups

As promised in Chapter 6, here are some of my favorite soup recipes.

World's Best Minestrone

The secret to making the world's best minestrone is to roast the vegetables first. It tastes great and is incredibly healthy. Veggies, beans and pasta make this minestrone a meal in a bowl.

Soup ingredients

2 tbsp. olive oil
1 large fennel bulb, cored and coarsely chopped
3 garlic cloves, chopped
1 large red pepper, coarsely chopped
3 large carrots, sliced (not too thin)
1 large onion, coarsely chopped
2 medium zucchini, quartered lengthwise, then sliced (not too thin)
1 summer squash, sliced the same as zucchini
1 28-oz. can of diced tomatoes
1 15-oz. can undrained cannelloni beans
1 15-oz. can undrained red kidney beans
3/4 cup uncooked ditalini (or other small pasta)
4 cups chicken stock/broth (may need more)
2 tsp. Mrs. Dash Italian Medley
1/4 cup grated parmesan cheese
Salt & pepper to taste

Directions

-Preheat oven to 375 F.

-In a large bowl, toss fennel, red pepper, carrots, onion, zucchini, summer squash and garlic with olive oil, salt and pepper. Spread on baking sheet. Roast veggies 30 minutes, stirring around every 10 minutes.

-While veggies cook, bring pot of salted water to boil, add pasta and cook al dente, drain, rinse and set aside.

-When veggies are done, transfer them to a large soup pot. Add diced tomatoes, cannelloni and red beans with their liquid, chicken stock/broth and Italian spices. Bring to boil, reduce heat and simmer 30 minutes. Give it an occasional stir.

-Add pasta and Parmesan. Reduce heat to low and let it sit for a half-hour or so to blend flavors. Thin with extra broth or water.

-Season with salt and pepper to taste.

Recipe makes about 8 pints.

Cajun Corn Chowder

Wild rice gives this creamy soup added texture and a nutty taste to go along with lip-smacking Cajun spices.

Soup ingredients

2 tbsp. olive oil
1 lb. package frozen corn, thawed
1 medium-large onion, coarsely chopped
3-4 medium carrots, coarsely chopped
3-4 garlic cloves, chopped
3/4 cup wild rice
1/4 lb. kielbasa sausage (or andouille), quartered lengthwise, then sliced to make little wedges
8 cups chicken stock or broth
1 tsp. each oregano, thyme, basil & cumin
1/4 tsp. cayenne pepper
1 12-oz. can fat-free evaporated milk
Salt & pepper to taste

Directions

-Bring 2 1/2 cups chicken stock to boil, add wild rice. Reduce heat to medium-low, cover and cook 40 minutes, until rice is almost tender, stirring occasionally.
-Heat oil in a large soup pot over medium heat, add onions, carrots and garlic. Cook 5 minutes, stirring frequently. Add sausage, oregano, thyme, basil, cumin and cayenne. Cook 5 minutes longer.
-Add four cups chicken broth, bring to boil, then reduce heat, cover (not too tightly) and simmer 20 minutes.

-While that is cooking, put 3/4 lb. corn in blender, add enough chicken stock to nearly cover corn and blend. Result should be about as thick as a good milkshake.
-Add wild rice and corn mixture to soup along with remaining 1/4 lb. corn. Continue simmering 15 minutes, then reduce heat to low, add 8 to 12 oz. evaporated milk and let flavors blend for 15-30 minutes.
-Season with salt and pepper to taste.

Recipe makes about 8 pints

Spicy Shrimp & Clam Chowder

How do you improve on nice,
spicy Manhattan clam chowder?
Just add shrimp!

Soup ingredients
2 tbsp. olive oil
1 large onion, chopped
3 stalks celery, chopped
½ green pepper, chopped
2-3 garlic cloves, minced
1 large peeled potato, cubed
28 oz. can diced tomatoes (or 1 box Pom)
3 6½-oz. cans chopped clams
8-oz. bottle clam juice
2 cups shrimp stock – see recipe below
¾ pound raw shrimp
½ tsp. dried thyme
1 capful liquid crab oil or dash of cayenne pepper*
Salt and pepper to taste

*Best to add crab boil/cayenne a little at a time and taste test until you get desired level of heat.

Directions
-Peel shrimp, boil shells gently for 15 minutes or so in 2-3 cups water to make a shrimp stock. If you don't want to bother, just use water.
-In a large soup pot, heat oil over medium heat and sauté onion, celery, green pepper and garlic for 10 minutes, stirring frequently.
-Add juice from clam cans, bottled clam juice, potato, thyme and crab boil or cayenne pepper. Bring to boil,

lower heat and simmer covered 20 minutes.
-Bring to boil, add shrimp and cook 5 minutes.
-Turn down heat, add tomatoes, clams and enough shrimp stock/water to get right consistency.
-Simmer 5 minutes.
-Season with salt and pepper to taste.

Recipe makes about 8 pints.

Split Pea Soup

When I was a kid, my mom was famous for her "hot dog" soup, which I refused to even try because didn't eat any soup. I was in my late teens before I even chanced a sip – and have been hooked ever since. My mom, Nomi, got the recipe from her mother-in-law, my Nana Mary, but it requires two days of cooking. My recipe is simpler and quicker and still very tasty because I use their trick of substituting kosher hot dogs for the traditional ham.

Soup ingredients

1 tsp. olive oil
1 medium onion, finely chopped
3-4 garlic cloves, minced
3-4 medium carrots, sliced 1/4-inch thick
20 oz. split peas, rinsed and drained
3-4 kosher hot dogs, quartered lengthwise, then sliced to make little wedges
12 cups organic chicken broth or stock
1/2 tsp. pepper
1 tsp. sea salt (or more to taste)

Directions

-In a soup pot, heat olive oil at medium heat, add chopped onions, sliced carrots and minced garlic and sauté until they soften and start to caramelize (5 to 10 minutes).
-Add rinsed split peas and toss around to mix with other ingredients.
-Add chicken stock, salt and pepper. Cover (slightly ajar) and boil vigorously 30 minutes.

- Turn down heat. Add hot dog wedges and simmer 30 minutes or until peas are broken down into mush.
-Add water or broth to thin as necessary.
-Season with salt and pepper to taste.

Recipe makes 6-7 pints.

Kitty's Creamy Crab Bisque

During the War of 1812, a lady named Kitty Knight convinced a British admiral to spare her house when the Red Coats invaded the eastern shore of Chesapeake Bay and burned most of Georgetown, Maryland, to the ground. Although Kitty was from a prominent family and was said to have danced with George Washington at the Continental Congress in Philadelphia, stubborn rumors persist that her house in this scenic town on the banks of Sassafras River was a brothel. It still stands today as an inn and restaurant with its own website that proclaims, "The historic Kitty Knight has been making special memories for generations." No doubt. My childhood memories of the Kitty Knight House are of creaky wooden stairs, bathroom fixtures that seemed straight out of the early 19th century and the most amazing soup. My mom got the recipe and couldn't believe how simple it was to make.
Neither will you.

Soup ingredients

6 11.5-oz. cans Campbell's green pea soup
4 11.5-oz. cans Campbell's tomato soup
4 6-oz. cans crab meat
1 5-oz. can evaporated milk (whole, 2% or fat-free)
1/2 cup sherry
1-2 tsp. liquid crab boil
2-3 cups water

Directions

-In a large soup pot, combine Campbell's pea and tomato soups, fluid from the crabmeat cans and 1

cup water. Turn heat to medium and use whisk to combine pea soup and tomato soup. This may take 10-15 minutes because the pea soup is very gelatinous, but you want the soup to heat up slowly or it will burn at the bottom of the pot. Add water as needed to produce a creamy base.
-When soup is lump-free and hot, add 1 tsp. crab boil. Stir in.
-Add crabmeat. Stir in.
-Add sherry. Stir in.
-Add evaporated milk. Stir in.
-Add more crab boil. (1/2 to 1 tsp. depending on how hot you like it. Taste test to get it right.)
-Add water to get desired consistency, if necessary.
-Reduce heat to low and let sit for a half-hour or so, stirring occasionally with wooden spatula, scraping bottom of pot to keep from burning.

Recipe makes 9-plus pints.

New England Clam Chowder

OK, it's easy to make a delicious New England clam chowder using heavy cream, because all that fat gives it great taste and texture. This soup achieves all that with just a fraction of the saturated fat. And using tender whole mussels instead of chewy clams will give your jaw a break.

Soup ingredients

1-2 Tbs. olive oil
4-5 strips cooked 'n' crumbled bacon
2-3 onions, chopped
3 medium red potatoes, peeled and cubed
4 stalks celery chopped
4 garlic cloves, minced
3 6-oz. cans minced clams
1 lb. mussels fresh (steamed and shelled) or frozen (thawed)
8 oz. clam broth
1 pint fat-free half & half
1 Tbs. flour
8 oz. milk
2 bay leaves
Sea salt, pepper and a touch of cayenne (or 1/2 cap liquid crab boil) if you want a little kick

Directions

-In a large soup pot, heat olive oil and add onions, celery and garlic, and cook on medium 5 minutes or so.
-Add potatoes, stir fry till potatoes start to brown.
-Add clam broth, fluid from canned clams, crumbled bacon, bay leaves, sea salt, pepper and cayenne (or

crab boil).
-Bring to boil, reduce heat and simmer at least 20 minutes.
-Whisk together half and half, milk and flour. Add to pot and cook at medium-high for a couple of minutes.
-Add canned clams plus clam meat or mussels and cook on medium for a couple of minutes while stirring - not too long or else the clams will get overcooked and rubbery.
-Add water or clam broth if needed to get good consistency.

Recipe makes 5-6 pints.

Asian Delight

Nora had some bok choy and napa cabbage left over from a stir fry, so I used it for an Asian-style soup. Shrimp, shitake mushrooms, ginger root and lo mein noodles make for great texture and taste, with a little kick from red pepper flakes.

Soup ingredients

2 tbsp. olive oil
4 scallions, sliced
3-4 garlic cloves, chopped
2 inches ginger root, peeled and sliced thin or grated
6-8 oz. shitake mushrooms caps, sliced
1 small bok choy, shredded
1/2 medium napa cabbage, shredded
1 lb. raw shrimp, cut in half
6 cups chicken stock/broth
8 oz. clam juice or 1-2 cups shrimp stock (see recipe)
4 oz. Chinese lo mein noodles, broken up
2 tsp. crushed red pepper flakes
Salt & pepper to taste

Directions

-Peel shrimp, boil shells gently in 2 cups water to make a shrimp stock. If you don't want to bother, use clam juice.
-In a large soup pot, heat olive oil at medium-high, add mushrooms, bok choy, napa cabbage, ginger, garlic and red pepper flakes. Stir around for a minute or so.
-Add chicken broth, shrimp stock or clam juice, cover and bring to boil.

-Add shrimp and noodles, boil 3 minutes.
-Add scallions, boil 2 minutes more.
-Turn off heat. Let sit 3 minutes.
-Season with salt and pepper to taste.

NOTE: Don't cook this one too long or the noodles and veggies will turn mushy.

Recipe makes about 6-7 pints.

Italian Wedding Soup

Spinach, kale, grass-fed beef and barley make this soup as nutritious as it is delicious.

Soup ingredients
2 tsp. olive oil
2 leeks, white and green parts, chopped
3-4 scallions or 1 yellow onion, chopped
4 medium carrots, chopped
2 ribs celery, chopped
5 garlic cloves, minced
12 cups organic chicken broth or stock
2 bay leaves
3/4 cup barley*
6 oz. baby spinach
4 oz. kale, center stem removed, leaves chopped
meatballs (see recipe below)
Italian blend spices
sea salt, pepper

*Barley: Follow directions on packaging but cook just 1/2 recommended time so that barley will absorb the rest from the soup stock.

Meatball ingredients
1 lb. grass-fed ground beef
1 small onion
2 garlic cloves
1 egg
bread crumbs

1 tsp. fine sea salt
1 tsp. pepper

Directions

-In a soup pot, heat olive oil at medium heat, add leeks, scallions/onion, carrots, celery and garlic and sauté until they soften and start to caramelize (5 to 10 minutes).
-Add healthy sprinkling of Italian seasoning (like Mrs. Dash) and mix in.
-Add chicken broth/stock and bay leaves, bring to boil. Lower heat, cover and simmer 30 minutes.
-Add barley, simmer another 10 minutes
-Add meatballs, simmer another 10 minutes.
-Add spinach and kale, simmer 5 minutes more.
-Add broth or water to reach desired consistency.
-Season with salt and pepper to taste.

Meatballs

With your hands, mix all ingredients except Panko crumbs in a large bowl. Add Panko until the right consistency for forming meatballs is achieved. Make small meatballs (1 lb. should yield at least 50) and bake at 350 degrees for 10 minutes (they'll finish cooking in the soup).

Recipe makes about 8 pints.

Appendix II
Cheat Sheet

For those of you who are either not interested in reading the whole book or don't want to continually leaf through it to remember how I manage to drink a lot of beer and not gain weight, here's what I do in a nutshell:

- **Understand the dangers of alcohol.** The Demon is addictive and destructive. Drinking more than two 5 percent ABV beers a day has been proven to be harmful to health and longevity for men, and that number drops to one for women. Since I overindulge, I try to do many other things to help compensate.
- **Be proactive.** I've learned about how the body works and stay vigilant for signs that something is wrong. When I see a healthcare provider, I am armed with knowledge about the condition so I can discuss it as it relates to my individual case. While I understand doctors and other professionals have more knowledge and training than I do, I possess knowledge about my own body that they don't have. So I work with them rather than just blindly following their recommendations.
- **Diet.** I don't count calories but am always aware of what I am putting in my mouth. During the week, I try to eat very healthily. That means an Isagenix protein shake for breakfast, homemade soup and fruit for lunch, and a sensible, nutrient-dense

dinner that usually includes a green salad, lean protein and veggies (often roasted). If I have a starch, such as rice or pasta, I use whole grain. On weekends, I eat whatever I want but try not to be stupid about it.

- **Liquid refreshment.** Besides beer, I waste very few calories on fluids. That means almost no soda, fruit juices or sports drinks. My default drink is purified water. If I want some flavor, I drink green ice tea with a little honey, ice coffee with just a splash of cream, or sparkling water with natural flavors.
- **Intermittent fasting.** I fast one day a week, usually from Sunday night to Tuesday morning, drinking only water and a very low-calorie cleansing concoction. It gives my body some time to do maintenance and repair and, to some degree, is like hitting a physiological reset button. Since I started doing it nearly a decade ago, my weight has remained stable.
- **January beer fast.** A month-long abstinence from alcohol is much more difficult for me than a day without eating, but I feel it's vitally important for my body. Besides giving my liver and other organs a break, I lose a few pounds and save a couple hundred bucks on beer.
- **Exercise.** I ride my bike for 30-45 minutes every weekday morning, including 1-2 days of high intensity interval training (HIIT). I spend about 45 minutes a day stretching out, including using a foam roller and inversion table. I also do some body weight resistance training in the form of push-ups, planks, deep knee bends and other calisthenics, often to break up long periods of sitting in a chair by a computer.

- **Lifestyle.** Along with diet and exercise, it's important to sleep well, nurture social connections and set aside some time every day to unwind. I use melatonin spray to help regulate my circadian rhythm to get a good night's sleep, pal around with rugby friends and others, and get close to nature and my evening beer by sitting by a turtle pen at my home. I also practice Earthing, walking around barefoot a lot to pick up negatively charged particles from the Earth to neutralize damaging, positively-charged free radicals in my body.
- **Anti-aging.** I take five "supplements" (pterostilbene, nicotinamide mononucleotide, astaxanthin, curcumin and carnosine) that together support all seven functions of cells. Keeping cells healthy is the key to longevity and overall health, and will no doubt extend your beer drinking years. Recommended reading: *The Kaufmann Protocol: Why We Age and How to Stop It.*

Special Bonus
The Body by the Numbers

Just so you know what you're made of...
Here's a reprint of a magazine article I wrote.

What a piece of work is man!

Shakespeare's words never ring truer than when you look at the amazing, incredible conglomeration of protoplasm known as the human body. Our bones are as strong as steel at one-third the weight, our stomach acid is potent enough to dissolve razor blades, and apart from its flammability, human hair is virtually indestructible.

But it's the numbers that are really mind-boggling - and that's saying a lot considering our brains perform 38 billion operations a second. Even at that rate, it would still take 5.8 billion years to count all of the 7 octillion atoms in our bodies.

And yet, we aren't really all there. A whopping 90 percent of the cells in our bodies are bacteria, not human. We have some 20 billion bacteria living in our mouths alone, more than double the number of humans on Earth. And our belly buttons harbor 67 different species of bacteria.

Of the human cells, our brains are no doubt the most remarkable collection. Despite our penchant for forgetting where we left our car keys, the brain is like a super-computer with estimates of storage capacity hitting as high as 1,000 terabytes. The 3-pound organ has 100 billion cells, and a piece of brain tissue the size of a sand grain contains 100,000 neurons and a billion synapses, all in constant communication. When we stub a toe, the impulse races to the brain at speeds up to 170 mph. And don't take offense if someone calls you dimwitted, seeing how the brain runs on the same amount of energy as a 10-watt lightbulb.

Of course, we don't have to think about our heart beating, which it does 100,000 times a day. The tireless muscle pumps 48 million gallons of blood in a lifetime, passing through about 70,000 miles of blood vessels, more than enough length to the circle the globe twice.

Speaking of length, if you unraveled all the DNA in a human, the strand would stretch to the sun and back 300 times. Meanwhile, 99 percent of humans' genetic makeup is identical, just slightly above the 97 percent we share with chimpanzees.

Our sensory organs are nothing to sneeze at, even though sneezes move air at up to 100 mph. Our noses can detect 50,000 different scents and, yes, women's sniffers tend to be more sensitive than those of men. That can work to a guy's advantage seeing how people pass gas an average of 13 times a day. Our eyes are equivalent to a 576-megapixel camera and can perceive 10 million different colors. We blink them 430 million times, meaning that we spend about 1.2 waking years of our lives in the dark.

Babies are born with 300 bones, but many fuse as we age, which is why adults have 206. About a quarter of them are in our feet, which also house 500,000 sweat glands. They produce about a pint of perspiration a day, a good reason for leaving those workout sneakers outside. In total, we excrete 15,000 quarts of sweat in a lifetime and cry 72 quarts of tears. The liver may be the hardest working organ in the body, performing some 500 functions. The kidneys process 13 million gallons of blood in a lifetime, producing 8,000 gallons of urine. The bladder holds between 150 and 230 cubic inches of urine, but we feel the urge to go before it's even half full. We also produce a quart of mucus a day, not to mention 6,500 gallons of saliva in a lifetime.

Our bodies are 60 percent water, but we have enough iron to make a 3-inch nail and enough carbon to fill 9,000 lead pencils. We also have .2 milligrams of gold in our blood. Still, the bottom line is that you could buy all of the basic elements in the human body for under $5.

Acknowledgments

I'd like to acknowledge everyone who helped with this book, but due to the amount of beer I've consumed over a lifetime, I can't remember their names.

Just kidding. The first one on my list is my lovely wife Nora, who always supports whatever I do, even when it is utterly screwed up. Second is Glen, my charming, handsome, clever and loving son, and go-to proofreader. My brother Steve also proofed the book, so cheers to him even though he doesn't drink beer. Thanks to my mom Nomi for her undying love and support, as well as shaming me into my first month-long beer fast. And to keep it in the family, this book may never have come to be without my other brother Rick telling me about his pal John Eaton's beer diet.

I owe gratitude to the really smart people who have shared with me their vast knowledge about health and well-being, particularly Dr. Sandra Kaufmann, Dr. James Galvin, Bill Faloon, Matt Kaeberlein, Dr. Jason Burke, Dr. Corey Cameron and Dr. Jason Fung. This information came to me primarily through interviews I conducted with them (and the other experts quoted) for various articles through the years and not in regards to beer's impact on the body. They have not directly participated in the creation of this book, nor have they reviewed the material or in any way endorsed how I've incorporated that information in this book.

I'd like to thank John Eaton for *his* beer diet, and being a good enough sport to let me tell the world about it. And I can't forget my many rugby teammates (and opponents), with whom I've shared some of my happiest beer-drinking times, and continue to do so.

Thanks to everyone who has helped promote this book, including Tom Madden, Adrienne Mazzone, Dilara Tuncer and the gang at TransMedia Group, my new Dutch pal Jos Struik, and the members of my "Book Launch Team." And huge thanks to two supremely talented individuals, cover illustrator and designer Jason Robinson, and sports photographer Tom DiPace, who snapped the amazing shot of me in action on the back cover.

I'd also like to recognize the visionaries who carved the craft beer industry out of a rather barren landscape of mostly taste-challenged lagers, as well as the Ryan Sentzes of the world, who continue to innovate and boldly go where beer brewers have not gone before. And, finally, thanks to the late Dolly Neuman and anyone else who has ever given me beer.

Cheers!

Made in the USA
Columbia, SC
18 August 2023